龍岡会の考える介護のあたりまえ
豊かに生きる、地域で暮らす

大森順方

Tatsuoka Group's Standard in Human Care
A Rich, Full Life, Lived in the Community

Nobumasa Ohmori

JN146388

はじめに

「明るいニッポンをつくるのは敬老化から」「笑顔の中から誇りが見られる」
最初の老人保健施設『龍岡』を建ててから今年で丸20年。以降、『浅草』『ワセダ』『千壽』……と、必要とされる地域へ、ときを空けずに介護施設を建ててきました。
介護施設のタイプとして老人保健施設を選んだのは、高齢者にとって一番のQOLは「住み慣れた自宅で暮らし続けること」という思いから。必要とするときだけ施設を利用し、元気になったら自宅に戻れる仕組みをつくりたいと考えました。
「龍岡会」は、祖父と父の2代にわたり、医師として、地域に根ざした医療を続けてきました。私の代で介護サービスも加わりましたが、土台となる理念はずっと変わっていません。

　　それぞれのゲストにふさわしい十人十色のケアー
　　心の癒される誠心誠意のケアー
　　いつでも信頼される生涯安心のケアー

光と風を感じるようにと、こだわり続けた空間設計の中で、3つの"龍岡イズム"が広がります。
高齢化のスピードは目を見張るものがあり、国が制度で支えていくには限界があります。「龍岡会」では、現状の介護の限界に目を向け、まっしろな状態から、高齢者が本当に望む暮らしやサービスを提供しています。
優しい心を持つスタッフが提供するケアーは、優しい施設をつくります。その思いや取り組みは地域社会へと広がり、平和な日本、そして安寧な世界を築くことにつながるでしょう。
この本を手に取った人に、少しでもわたしたちの思いが伝わり、共に明るいニッポンの未来をつくる同志になっていただけることを願います。

2016年7月
医療法人社団 龍岡会
社会福祉法人 龍岡会
理事長 大森順方

Preface

"The building of a bright Japan starts with respect for the aged" "Pride shows in smiling faces"
This year marks a full 20 years since the founding of our first geriatric health care services facility, "Tatsuoka." Since then, we have continued to construct health care facilities as and where they have been needed; "Asakusa," "Waseda," "Senju"...
As to why we chose to build geriatric health care services facilities, this came from the idea that for the elderly, the most important factor in QOL (quality of life) is "Being able to continue living in your own home, where you are most comfortable." We wanted to create a system whereby the elderly would make use of the facility only when necessary, and go back to their own home when their condition improved. Over two generations, my father and grandfather worked as physicians, providing community-based medical treatment. To this I have added health care services, but the underlying principles of the Tatsuoka Group remain unchanged.

 Guest Oriented Care
 Hearty Care
 After Care

These three principle of "Tatsuokaism"(Tatsuoka-style care) are tangible throughout the spatial design we have always insisted on, in much the same way as one feels light and fresh air.
The speed at which our society is aging is quite breathtaking, and there are limits to what government systems can do. At the Tatsuoka Group, we focus our attention on the limitations in the current health care situation, and with no preconceptions offer the elderly the lifestyle and services they truly desire. The care provided by a kind-hearted staff makes the facility compassionate. If this way of thinking and acting can spread to the local community, surely it will lead to the building of a harmonious Japan and eventually a more tranquil world.
I hope that this booklet will help you understand something of our aspirations, and that you will join us in working together to create a bright future for Japan.

Nobumasa Ohmori
Chairperson
Medical Corporation Tatsuoka
Social Welfare Corporation Tatsuoka
July 2016

目次

はじめに ——— 2
大森順方

沿革 ——— 8

1章　わたしたちの実践 ——— 9

山手線環内で初の老人保健施設の誕生

伝えていくものと変えていくもの

グレーゾーンにあえて踏み込む

家族の風景を描く

徹底した現場主義

夢を持って生きよう

高齢化は"問題"ではない

2章　龍岡会を伝える30のキーワード ——— 25

① 図面上にだけあるライン
② ノックがいらない関係
③ あえてシロ
④ むきだしの美
⑤ 門構え（ファサード）からいいものを
⑥ 壁一面の大きな窓
⑦ 窓から先の風景も考える
⑧ 柔らかい光の演出
⑨ 壁に同化するクリーンルーム
⑩ 一方通行のエレベーター
⑪ 押しても引いても開くドア
⑫ 長生きする素材
⑬ ウッドデッキでBBQ
⑭ 静の空間、動の空間
⑮ 近すぎず、遠すぎず
⑯ 北欧家具のシークレット
⑰ どこにでも椅子
⑱ 子どもあつかいしないサイン
⑲ 湯船に浸かるのはニッポンの文化
⑳ おいしさは脳で感じる

3章 インタビュー スタッフの取り組み ──── 89

㉑ 食の30秒ルール

㉒ 好きなものを、みんなで一緒に

㉓ 介護食のイノベーション

㉔ ハーティーミール®

㉕ スタッフは芸術家

㉖ ケアーサイエンス®＝答えを出す

㉗ 小さな夢を叶えるプロジェクト

㉘ 外出のもうひとつの狙い

㉙ 地域への架け橋

㉚ 介護に国境はない

介護部の取り組み
一生青春、一生感動

介護部の取り組み
"夢見がち"なところと、"タフ"なところと

相談部の取り組み
施設の要、ヒューマンコーディネーター

プロジェクト部の取り組み
スタッフの満足度を高める仕掛けづくり

栄養部の取り組み
思い出の料理をもう一度

アート部の取り組み
人生にアートは欠かせない

アート部の取り組み
大手ホテルでの展覧会

医療への取り組み
暮らしを支える町の診療所

スタッフの海外研修
五感で学ぶ

施設紹介 ──── 121

龍岡介護老人保健施設

浅草介護老人保健施設

櫻川介護老人保健施設

神石介護老人保健施設

千壽介護老人保健施設

千壽グループホーム

ワセダグループホーム

青葉ヒルズ（特別養護老人ホーム）

Preface ———— 2

Nobumasa Ohmori

History ———— 8

Chapter 1 What We Do ———— 9

The Birth of the First Geriatric Health Care Services Facility
within the Yamanote Line Area

Things We Continue and Things We Change

Venturing into a Gray Zone

Creating a Family Atmosphere

A Hands-on Approach in Everything

Hold on to Your Dreams

Aging is Not a "Problem"

Chapter 2 30 Key Phrases: The Essence of the Tatsuoka Group ———— 25

① No Partitions
② No Knocking Required
③ Choosing White
④ Undressed Beauty
⑤ High Quality from the Front Gate
⑥ Wall-sized Windows
⑦ Scenery Beyond the Window
⑧ Soft, Dramatic Light
⑨ Invisible Clean Room
⑩ One-way Elevators
⑪ Our Special Doors
⑫ Long-living Materials
⑬ Barbecue Parties
⑭ Stillness and Motion
⑮ Not Too Close, Not Too Far
⑯ The Magic of Scandinavian Furniture
⑰ Chairs Everywhere
⑱ Signs That are Simple, Not Childish
⑲ Soaking in the Bath:
   It's Part of Being Japanese

CONTENTS

(20) Umami is in the Mind

(21) The 30-second Rule for Hot Meals

(22) Sharing the Joys of Favorite Foods Together

(23) Innovative Human-care Food

(24) Hearty Meal®

(25) Staff Who are Artists

(26) Care Science® = Finding Answers

(27) Making Modest Dreams Come True

(28) The Other Goal of Outings

(29) Bridges to the Local Community

(30) No Borders in Human Care

Chapter 3 Interviews: Staff Endeavor ———— 89

Endeavor in the Care Department
Lifelong Youth, Lifelong Inspiration

Endeavor in the Care Department
Both "Visionary" and "Tough"

Endeavor in the Counseling Department
A Linchpin of the Facility: The Human Coordinator

Endeavor in the Projects Department
Developing Ways to Raise Staff Satisfaction

Endeavor in the Nutrition Department
A Taste of Nostalgia

Endeavor in the Art Department
Art is an Indispensable Part of Life

Endeavor in the Art Department
Exhibitions at Leading Hotels

Endeavor in Medical Care
The Town Clinic at the Center of Local Life

Overseas Staff Training
Learning Through the Five Senses

Facilities ———— 121

Tatsuoka Geriatric Health Care Services Facility

Asakusa Geriatric Health Care Services Facility

Sakuragawa Geriatric Health Care Services Facility

Kamiishi Geriatric Health Care Services Facility

Senju Geriatric Health Care Services Facility

Senju Group Home

Waseda Group Home

Aoba Hills (Special Nursing Home)

医療法人社団 龍岡会・社会福祉法人 龍岡会 沿革

1927年	4月	大森医院 開業
1993年	12月	医療法人社団 龍岡会 設立
1996年	3月	龍岡老人保健施設 開設
		（H12年介護保険法により龍岡介護老人保健施設に改称）
	4月	龍岡在宅介護支援センター 開設
	10月	龍岡訪問看護ステーション 開設
2000年	4月	龍岡ケアーマネイジメントセンター 開設
		メディケアーマネイジメントセンター 開設
		ナースケアーマネイジメントセンター 開設
		龍岡ヘルパーステーション 開設
2001年	4月	浅草介護老人保健施設 開設
2003年	4月	龍岡訪問リハビリテーション 開設
		浅草訪問リハビリテーション 開設
2005年	4月	櫻川介護老人保健施設 開設
		櫻川訪問リハビリテーション 開設
		櫻川ケアーマネイジメントセンター 開設
		（※ナースケアーマネイジメントセンターを名称変更）
		櫻川ヘルパーステーション 開設
2006年	4月	龍岡在宅介護支援センター 法改正により、
		本富士地域包括支援センター（龍岡予防支援事業所）に改変
	7月	ワセダグループホーム 開設
	10月	メディケアーマネイジメントセンター、
		龍岡ケアーマネイジメントセンターに統合廃止
2007年	12月	社会福祉法人 龍岡会 設立
2009年	4月	青葉ヒルズ（特別養護老人ホーム）開設
2010年	4月	神石介護老人保健施設 開設
2013年	4月	千壽介護老人保健施設 開設
		千壽訪問看護ステーション 開設
		千壽グループホーム 開設
2015年	5月	千壽訪問看護ステーションを
		龍岡訪問看護ステーション千壽サテライトステーションに改変

History of Medical Corporation Tatsuoka / Social Welfare Corporation Tatsuoka

1927	Apr.	Opening of the Ohmori Clinic
1993	Dec.	Foundation of Medical Corporation Tatsuoka
1996	Mar.	Opening of the Tatsuoka Geriatric Health Care Facility
		(Renamed the Tatsuoka Geriatric Health Care Services Facility in 2000, in accordance with the Long-Term Care Insurance Act)
	Apr.	Opening of the Tatsuoka Home Care Support Center
	Oct.	Opening of the Tatsuoka Visiting Nurse Station
2000	Apr.	Opening of the Tatsuoka Care Management Center
		Opening of the Medicare Management Center
		Opening of the Nurse Care Management Center
		Opening of the Tatsuoka Helper Station
2001	Apr.	Opening of the Asakusa Geriatric Health Care Services Facility
2003	Apr.	Opening of Tatsuoka Visiting Rehabilitation
		Opening of Asakusa Visiting Rehabilitation
2005	Apr.	Opening of the Sakuragawa Geriatric Health Care Services Facility
		Opening of Sakuragawa Visiting Rehabilitation
		Opening of the Sakuragawa Care Management Center
		(*Name changed to Nurse Care Management Center)
		Opening of the Sakuragawa Helper Station
2006	Apr.	Due to an amendment to the law, change from the Tatsuoka Home Care Support Center to the Motofuji Community General Support Center/ Tatsuoka Caring Prevention Support Office
	Jul.	Opening of the Waseda Group Home
	Oct.	Discontinuance of the Medicare Management Center and integration into the Tatsuoka Care Management Center
2007	Dec.	Foundation of Social Welfare Corporation Tatsuoka
2009	Apr.	Opening of the Aoba Hills (Special Nursing Home)
2010	Apr.	Opening of the Kamiishi Geriatric Health Care Services Facility
2013	Apr.	Opening of the Senju Geriatric Health Care Services Facility
		Opening of the Senju Visiting Nurse Station
		Opening of the Senju Group Home
2015	May.	Change from the Senju Visiting Nurse Station to the Tatsuoka Visiting Nurse Station Senju Satellite Station

1章 わたしたちの実践

Chapter 1　What We Do

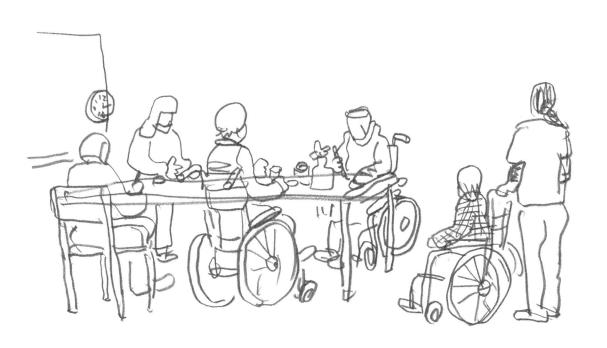

山手線環内で初の老人保健施設の誕生

「1996年、山手線環内で初の老人保健施設の誕生―」。都内ではじめての高齢者施設の誕生は、新聞紙上をにぎわせました。当時は介護保険制度の施行前、老人ホームは"暗い"というマイナスイメージが根強く残り、それは人里離れた場所にあるものだという考えで、都会に建てる発想などなかった頃です。そもそも老人保健施設とは、入所者（ゲスト）が元気になって在宅に戻ることを目標に、個々に合ったケアーを提供するための施設。そうであるならば、住み慣れた土地にあるのが道理のはず。私がまず目指したのは、"養老院（身寄りのない高齢者を収容して保護する施設）"からの脱却でした。

人々の意識にこびりついた老人ホームのイメージを変えるための私のアイデアは、これまでとはすべて"逆の発想"で進んでいくということ。公共性のある建物でもここまでできるということを、まずは自分が証明しようと思いました。

その思いで突き進んできた集大成は、2009年に完成した特別養護老人ホーム『青葉ヒルズ』です。建築家と「一緒に美しいものをつくりましょう」と、建物の細部にわたり、自然の恵みを感じる斬新なデザインにこだわりました。なじみの土地で人生の最期まで、そして、美しい建物の中で尊厳を持って暮らせる住まい。私がスタートから一貫して目指していたものが、ようやく形になったのです。

The Birth of the First Geriatric Health Care Services Facility within the Yamanote Line Area

"1996, Birth of First Geriatric Health Care Services Facility in Yamanote Line Area" — the birth of the first care facility for the elderly in Tokyo received a lot of coverage in the press. At the time the long-term care insurance system had not yet come into being; there was still a very strong negative image attached to "nursing homes," as a gloomy place that belonged in some distant, desolate setting. It was a time when no one thought of building one in the city.

Essentially, a geriatric health care services facility is a facility that provides customized care with the aim of restoring residents (guests) to good health so that they can then return home. That being the case, it makes sense that the facility should be located close to the guest's home. My first goal was to shake off the image of "nursing homes" as an facility for the care and protection of old people with nowhere else to go.

My idea for changing this deeply-engrained image of the nursing home was to take an approach that was the opposite of everything that had gone before. I wanted to prove first of all how much could be achieved even in a building that was public by nature.

The culmination of pushing forward with this idea was Aoba Hills, a special nursing home for the aged that was completed in 2009. Working with the architect, I wanted to "make something beautiful together," and in every detail of the building we insisted on an innovative design that spoke of the bounty of nature. A place of residence where people can live till the end in the location they are used to — and live with dignity in a building of beauty. What I had been aiming for right from the beginning had at last taken shape.

伝えていくものと変えていくもの

「看板は出さない、紹介者のみ」。これは、龍岡会の前身である大森医院の院長（祖父）からの教え。理由は、クチコミこそが本当の評価だから。祖父は、午前中は診察、午後は往診という町医者でした。東京帝国大学付属病院に勤務していた頃は、「大森先生の診察には列ができる」と噂になるほど、地域に根ざした医療を率先して行っていました。

祖父は、患者さんにはとても厳しい人で「病気は医者が治すものではない、自分で治すものだ」と、常に説いていました。私が自立を支援するリハビリ施設をはじめようと思ったのも、こうした意識を継いでいるところがあるのかもしれません。また、龍岡会では食の取り組みを積極的に進めていますが、それは「食は上薬にして医薬は下薬なり」という父の思想から続いています。

大森医院から新たな一歩を踏み出した龍岡会では、治療の場から暮らしの場へと、提供する場所が変わりました。科学的な裏づけも技術開発も日進月歩の医療とは違い、すべてが未開の介護の世界。私はこの世界は、変えていかなければならないものがまだたくさんあると感じています。

まず私ができることは、介護の世界に医療のよい部分を取り入れること。Care Science®（介護を科学すること）や、教育やアートなど専門的な部署を明確に分けることで、日々のケアーに追われて見失いがちな、けれどけっして疎かにしてはいけない視点を確立することからはじめました。

Things We Continue and Things We Change

"No need for a signboard; by referral only." This was the doctrine of my grandfather who was the director of the Ohmori Clinic, the precursor to the Tatsuoka Group. His reason was that it is word-of-mouth that reflects one's true reputation. My grandfather was a general practitioner, performing medical examinations in the morning and making house calls in the afternoon. When he worked at the University of Tokyo Hospital, the rumor was that due to his popularity there was "always a queue of patients at Dr. Ohmori's office." He took the initiative in community-based health care.

My grandfather was very strict with his patients, always asserting that "Illness isn't something the doctor cures; only the patient can cure himself." It may be that the reason I wanted to open a rehabilitation facility that would help patients regain their independence has something to do with carrying on his ideas. And the active pursuit by the Tatsuoka Group of dietary excellence comes from my father's philosophy that "Good food is the best medicine; pharmaceuticals are secondary."

Moving on in a new direction from the Ohmori Clinic, the Tatsuoka Group offers a living space rather than a place of treatment. Unlike medical treatment, where there is rapid progress in both scientific corroboration and technological developments, the long-term care industry is not up-to-date with the latest developments in healthcare and social changes. I feel that there is much in this world that still needs to be changed.

What I can do first of all is incorporate the beneficial aspects of medicine into the world of long-term care. I started by establishing a perspective that tends to be lost sight of in the day-to-day task of providing care, yet is something that must not be overlooked, by making a clear distinction between Care Science® and specialist areas like education and arts.

グレーゾーンにあえて踏み込む

介護の世界では、現状維持できればよいという考えの元、変えるべきものがそのまま放置されていました。固定概念が強い世界の中で「もっとよりよいものに変えていきましょう！」と訴え続ける私は、その当時、異端児あつかいをされていたかもしれません。それでも、誰かが言わないといつまでも変化は起きません。

ゲストと一緒に外出をすることは、ゲストにとってリフレッシュや社会参加になるだけではなく、社会に向けて気づきを与える絶好の機会です。だから私は、「お台場に行って観覧車に乗るのは迷惑がかかるかも」とか、「国技館２階席の入口へ行くには、エスカレーターしかないから車椅子のゲストは連れて行けない」というネガティブな理由で、外出を躊躇することはしていません。

国技館に相撲観戦に行ったときは、大相撲協会に勤めている元力士たちを呼んで、ゲストを会場までおぶってもらいました。元力士もゲストもみんなが笑顔で、よい思い出になったと思います。

制度というものはリスクを避ける。でも制度的には問題になることでも、それがゲストのためになったり、社会にたいして伝えるべきニーズであれば、あえてリスクに踏み込む。実は、無知ゆえの不親切だったという発見も多く、確実に変わっていくことがあるのです。

Venturing into a Gray Zone

In the world of long-term care, things that should be changed have been left as they are, based on the idea that maintaining the status quo is a good thing. In a world where traditional practice persists, I was probably looked on at the time as an eccentric for my repeated insistence that we should "make changes for the better!" Still, if no one speaks out, nothing will ever change.

Escorting guests on trips outside is more than just a means of providing guests with stimulation or a chance to be social; it is a great opportunity to increase awareness of care for the aged in our society. This is why I do not let negative thoughts such as "It might be inconvenient for others if we go to Odaiba to ride on the Ferris wheel" or "We can't take guests in wheelchairs to the upper level seats in the Kokugikan, because there is no elevator" stop our guests from taking trips outside.

When we went to watch sumo at the Kokugikan, we got some former sumo wrestlers of the Japan Sumo Association to volunteer and carry our guests into the venue on their backs. Both the former wrestlers and our guests had smiles on their faces, and I think it is something they all look back on with great pleasure.

Risk avoidance and inertia always permeate any system. But even with something that the system sees as a risk, if it's to the benefit of a guest, or if it's a need that society needs to be made aware of, the risk should be taken. In many cases it will be found that what seems to be inconsiderate is actually the result of ignorance, the correction of which will lead to sure and positive change.

家族の風景を描く

龍岡会では、現在5つの介護老人保健施設を運営しています。介護老人保健施設は、その成り立ちから、在宅をベースにケアーを考えます。

それでも、様々な事情から自宅にもどることがむずかしい人がいます。これから高齢化を迎えるにあたり、そうした人も増えていくことになる。だから龍岡会では、三世代で住んでいた頃の大家族の温かみと知恵を、そのまま形にしたような施設のあり方を大事にしています。スタッフもテーブルに座り、会話を楽しみながら一緒に食事をします。

人生の先輩であるゲストから、スタッフが教わることはたくさんあります。その尊敬の気持ちがケアーをするのではなく、"させていただく"という思いを生むのでしょう。

『龍岡』に佇む、戦争も震災も耐えてきたシンボルの赤レンガ。建物であっても、日本が紡いできた文化を残していくことは忘れません。

人生の最期まで過ごせる『青葉ヒルズ』では、ユニットケアでアットホームなリビングルームをつくりました。10人単位の顔なじみの関係。そこでは毎食、家族の食卓を再現しています。

龍岡会で描かれるのは古きよき、大家族の風景。人はいかに老いるのか、どうやって死を迎えるのか。暮らしの中にそれぞれの人生が交差していると、みんなに労りの気持ちが浸透していくはずです。

Creating a Family Atmosphere

The Tatsuoka Group currently operates five geriatric health care services facilities. By its nature, such a facility is based on the idea of care centered on the home.

That said, there may be many reasons why it may be difficult for a person to return home. As the population continues to age, more and more people will find themselves in this situation. For this reason, the Tatsuoka Group places importance on being the kind of facility that maintains and preserves the warmth and good sense found in the extended family back in the days when it was common for three generations to live together under one roof. At mealtimes, staff members sit at the table with the guests, enjoying the conversation as they eat together.

There is a lot that the staff can learn from the guests, who have lived longer and seen more. It is this sense of respect that produces in the staff the feeling that they are not so much giving the guests care, rather they are privileged to be able to help them.

The symbolic red brick of Tatsuoka, survivors of both World War II and the Great Kanto Earthquake. It may only be a building, but we must not forget to pass on the culture woven by Japan.

What the Tatsuoka Group portrays is the atmosphere of the extended family of the good old days. How does a person age, in what way does that person face death? When people live their lives intersecting and interacting with each other, a feeling of compassion surely penetrates the fiber of each individual.

徹底した現場主義

私は毎日、ゲストが暮らす現場に足を運び、お顔を見て挨拶をして、生の声を聞いています。現場のスタッフから上がってきた意見も、できるだけフィルターを通さず、本人と話すようにします。それだけではなく、月に一度、各施設で実施する運営改善会議にも、すべて顔を出すようにしています。それは、「よい会社のトップは、会社の些細なことまで知っている」という考えから。常に、現場のための運営を考えられる頭でいたいのです。また、誰にたいしても平等に接するように心がけています。

スタッフは、基本的に新卒採用にしています。龍岡会のオリジナリティを大切にしたいので、既存の枠にとらわれず、まっさらな気持ちで介護の世界を見ることができる人を求めています。

そのため、年功序列にはけっしてせず、龍岡会の理念を理解して実践する人が、いつでもトップに立つことができる組織づくりを努めています。

デンマークの国会議員が視察に来たとき、「スタッフが本当に明るく働いている」と、目を丸くしていました。ルーティンワークな仕事をしていたら、きっと笑顔をなくしてしまうでしょう。

どこかの真似事をするのではなく、現場優先の環境の中で、自分たちで考え実践していく。その使命感と達成感が、スタッフにとって働きやすい職場になると信じています。

A Hands-on Approach in Everything

Every day I make my way to where our guests live, greet them face-to-face and listen to what they have to say. I make a point of discussing in person and directly with those concerned, the ideas and suggestions that have been brought up by staff members working with the guests. That is not all; I make a point of attending all of the management improvement meetings held once a month at each of our facilities. This comes from my conviction that in a good company, the person at the top knows everything about the company, right down to the smallest detail. I want to be at all times a leader who is capable of considering management in terms of what is best for those most affected. And I take care to treat everyone equally.

As a general rule, staff members are hired straight out of university. Because we want to preserve the originality of the Tatsuoka Group, we seek new recruits who are able to view the world of human care with an open mind, without stereotypes from past experience.

This means that seniority is not determined by length of service; we work hard to maintain a structure whereby anyone who understands and practices the principles of the Tatsuoka Group is always able to rise to the top.

When members of the Danish Parliament came to visit us, they were amazed at how cheerful the staff appeared to be as they went about their work. When work becomes nothing more than routine, that is surely when the smiles disappear.

Rather than simply going through the motions, our staff members think for themselves and act in an environment where their on-the-scene perspective has priority. I believe that it is that sense of mission and sense of achievement that creates a workplace that is supportive of the staff working there.

夢を持って生きよう

あるスタッフが、「夢見がちな施設であるところが好きです」と私に言いました。いつもスタッフたちには、口癖のように「夢を持って生きよう!」と話しています。

介護の現場は毎日が戦場です。食事、着替え、排泄、就寝準備など、目の前の対応に追われていると、あっという間に時間が過ぎてしまう。ゲストの命をお預かりする場なので、緊迫する場面もたくさん出てきます。さらに、よいケアーを提供しようとすればするほど、スタッフの労力はどんどん増えていく。

それでも龍岡会のスタッフたちは、ゲストにとってよいことは積極的に取り入れています。それは、ゲストの笑顔を見ることが、スタッフの夢でもあるからです。夢のある人は、何歳になっても輝いています。夢に向かって歩いているとき、人は輝き、喜びを感じるのです。

もちろん、日々の仕事に余裕がなければ、心に余裕は生まれません。そのために、暮らしにアートを取り入れたり、スタッフのケアーなど、龍岡会独自の取り組みに専門の担当者を配置しています。

小さな夢から一つひとつみんなで叶えていけば、いつの間にか大きな夢にまで手が届く。人を労り、思いやる心には、世界平和にもつながっていくほどの効力があるのです。

Hold on to Your Dreams

A staff member once said to me, "What I like about this place is that it is a facility where people can dream." I am always telling staff members to "Hold on to your dreams!"

In the front line of human care, every day is a battle. Meals, changing clothes, dealing with toilet needs, preparations for bedtime, etc., etc., — when you are caught up in dealing with what is in front of you, the time passes before you realize it. Because we are entrusted with the lives of our guests, things can often get tense. Added to that, the more we try to provide our guests with good human care, the greater the workload we impose on our staff.

Even so, the Tatsuoka Group staff members work diligently to do what is best for the guests. This is because seeing a smile on the face of a guest is what the staff member is working for. At whatever age, a person with a dream to work towards is radiant. It is in moving towards one's dream that a person feels that radiance, that joy.

Of course, if a person has no space to breathe in their day-to-day work, they will have no space to breathe mentally or spiritually. For this reason, we incorporate art into everyday life and employ professional staff to oversee the initiatives that are unique to the Tatsuoka Group, such as staff care, etc. If we fulfill one small dream after another, before we know it we will find ourselves within reach of a larger dream. The spirit of consideration and compassion for others has the power to contribute to world peace.

高齢化は"問題"ではない

日本では、団塊の世代がいよいよ人生の第4ステージに入っていきます。2020年には、4人に1人が65歳以上を迎えることになるでしょう。先進諸国に先駆けて高齢社会を迎えるため、世界中で日本の動向が注目されています。

世間では、高齢社会を"問題"として取り上げていますが、私は疑問を感じます。皆が平等に長生きできる平和な暮らしを望んできたのは、ほかでもない私たちなのです。

夢はいつまでも経っても色褪せない。ですが、それ以外の地球上にあるものはみな有限です。人類は長い歴史の中で、長生きすることを願いつづけてきました。そして今ようやく、「人生100年」といわれる長寿社会となり、長生きできる人々が増えました。

日本はこれまで、フェイタルなものにお金をかけてきませんでした。ですが、これからの時代は、老人が幸せになることがニッポンを明るくしていくことにつながるはず。それこそが、みんなの夢が叶った究極の未来の姿なのですから。

私たち龍岡会が立ち上げ当初から取り組んできた、利益を先に考えるのではなく、誠心誠意ゲストに尽くすこと。これは、22世紀に向けた、新しい社会のカタチになるかもしれません。

Aging is Not a "Problem"

In Japan in particular, the postwar baby boomers are now about to enter into what was traditionally called the fourth stage of life. By 2020, one in four of us will be aged 65 or over. Because we are the first of the developed countries to experience population aging, people all over the world are keeping a close eye on developments in Japan.

The world at large tends to look on the aging society as a "problem," but I question that view. After all, it is none other than we ourselves who have longed for a peaceful life in which everyone has a chance to enjoy a long life.

Everything else on this earth is finite but a dream never ever fades. Throughout his long history, Man has hoped and prayed for longevity. Today we have at last become a society of longevity, in which it is said that "the span of a man is 100 years," and a growing number of people are living longer lives.

In the past, the Japanese did not spend money on people who became very old. But in the era we are about to enter, surely having an elderly population that is happy will lead to a Japan where the future is bright for all; because that will ultimately shape the future in which all of our dreams will have come true. We render sincere and wholehearted service to our guests rather than putting profit first. This is what we at the Tatsuoka Group have put our efforts into from the start. This could be the shape of the new society that will take us into the 22nd century.

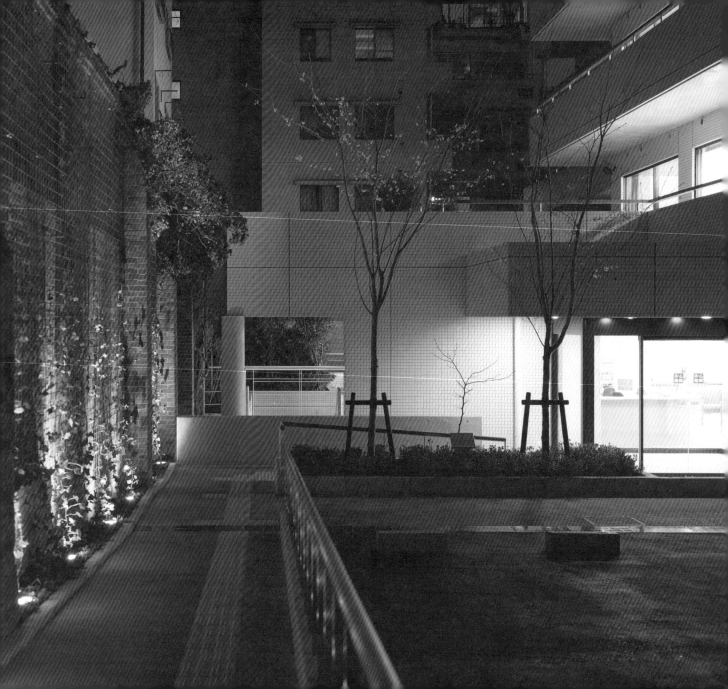

2章 龍岡会を伝える30のキーワード
Chapter 2 30 Key Phrases: The Essence of the Tatsuoka Group

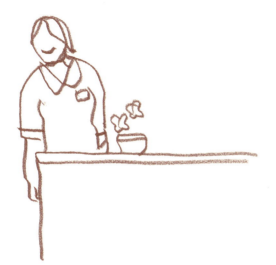

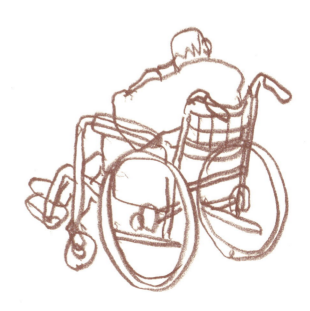

2章 龍岡会を伝える30のキーワード
Chapter 2　30 Key Phrases: The Essence of the Tatsuoka Group

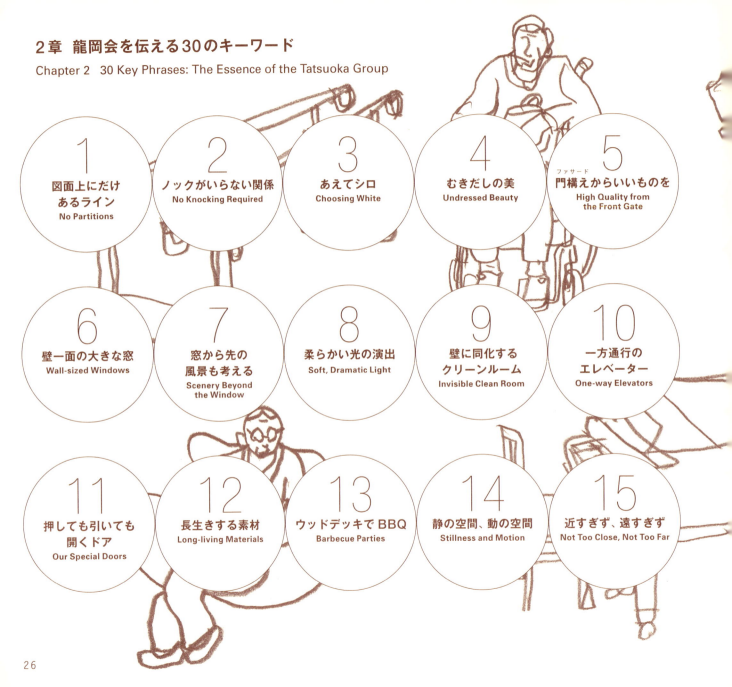

1. 図面上にだけあるライン
   No Partitions

2. ノックがいらない関係
   No Knocking Required

3. あえてシロ
   Choosing White

4. むきだしの美
   Undressed Beauty

5. 門構え(ファサード)からいいものを
   High Quality from the Front Gate

6. 壁一面の大きな窓
   Wall-sized Windows

7. 窓から先の風景も考える
   Scenery Beyond the Window

8. 柔らかい光の演出
   Soft, Dramatic Light

9. 壁に同化するクリーンルーム
   Invisible Clean Room

10. 一方通行のエレベーター
    One-way Elevators

11. 押しても引いても開くドア
    Our Special Doors

12. 長生きする素材
    Long-living Materials

13. ウッドデッキでBBQ
    Barbecue Parties

14. 静の空間、動の空間
    Stillness and Motion

15. 近すぎず、遠すぎず
    Not Too Close, Not Too Far

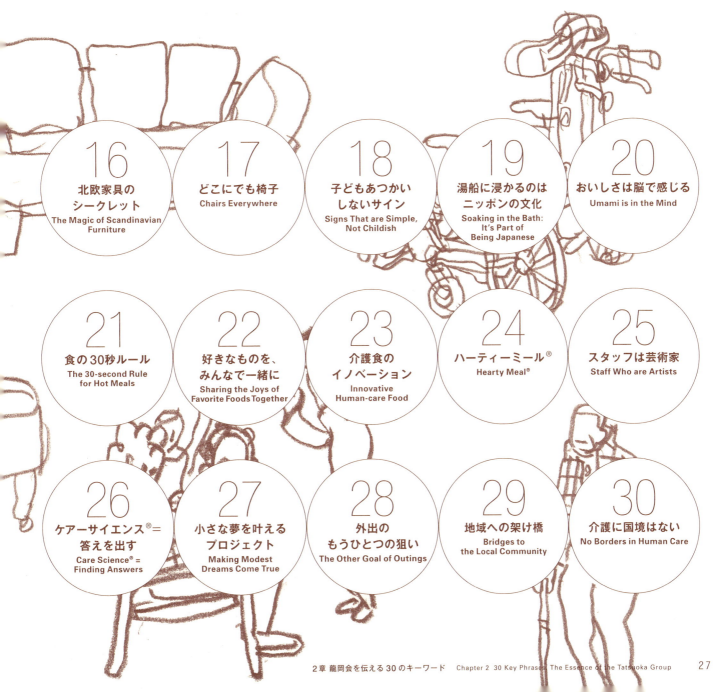

16	北欧家具のシークレット	The Magic of Scandinavian Furniture
17	どこにでも椅子	Chairs Everywhere
18	子どもあつかいしないサイン	Signs That are Simple, Not Childish
19	湯船に浸かるのはニッポンの文化	Soaking in the Bath: It's Part of Being Japanese
20	おいしさは脳で感じる	Umami is in the Mind
21	食の30秒ルール	The 30-second Rule for Hot Meals
22	好きなものを、みんなで一緒に	Sharing the Joys of Favorite Foods Together
23	介護食のイノベーション	Innovative Human-care Food
24	ハーティーミール®	Hearty Meal®
25	スタッフは芸術家	Staff Who are Artists
26	ケアーサイエンス®＝答えを出す	Care Science® = Finding Answers
27	小さな夢を叶えるプロジェクト	Making Modest Dreams Come True
28	外出のもうひとつの狙い	The Other Goal of Outings
29	地域への架け橋	Bridges to the Local Community
30	介護に国境はない	No Borders in Human Care

2章 龍岡会を伝える30のキーワード　Chapter 2　30 Key Phrases: The Essence of the Tatsuoka Group

図面上にだけあるライン
No Partitions

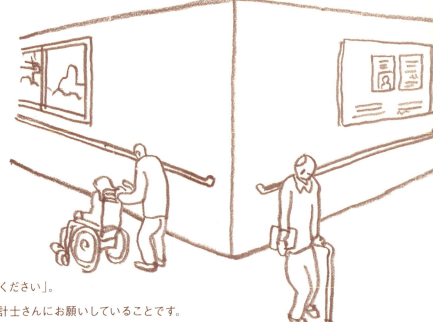

「共用部の仕切り(ライン)は、図面上だけにしてください」。
これは、新しい施設を設計するときに、最初に設計士さんにお願いしていることです。
みんなが集うリビングルームは、開放的で明るい空間にしたい。
玄関や各フロアーに一歩足を踏み入れると、視界を遮るものがないようなつくりを考えました。
そこでは毎日、朝の体操にはじまり、レクリエーションやコンサートなど、楽しいプログラムを開催。
仕切りがない空間では、音楽や笑い声がどこまでも響きわたります。

"These lines in the common area should only be on the blueprints."
When a new facility is being designed, this is my first request for the architect.
I want the living area where everyone gathers to be a bright and open space.
I feel that as soon as you step through the main entrance or get to a new floor, there shouldn't be anything blocking your view.
Every day, beginning with morning exercises, we have recreational activities, concerts, and other fun events in this space.
Not having any walls or partitions allows music and laughter to echo through the room.

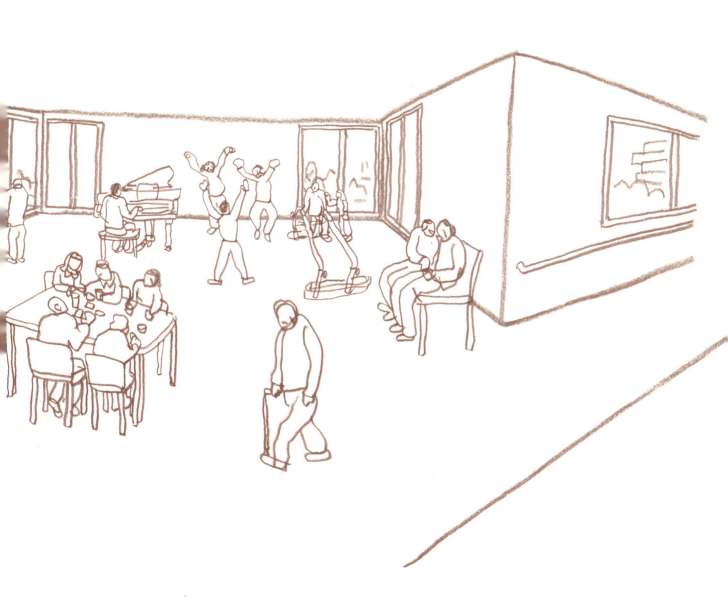

とかく介護の世界では、"お世話をしてあげている・してもらっている"関係に陥りやすいもの。

それでは、私がめざす風通しのよい関係は築けません。

最初の相談窓口となる玄関前の受付は、どの施設もオープンカウンターにしています。

これは、空間から仕掛ける"フラットな関係"づくりのプロローグ。

スタッフは受付業務だけではなく、相談作業もすべてそこで行います。

気軽に挨拶や声かけが習慣になると、スタッフもゲストの変化をすぐに察知でき

こちらから先に声をかけることができるのです。

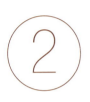

ノックがいらない関係
No Knocking Required

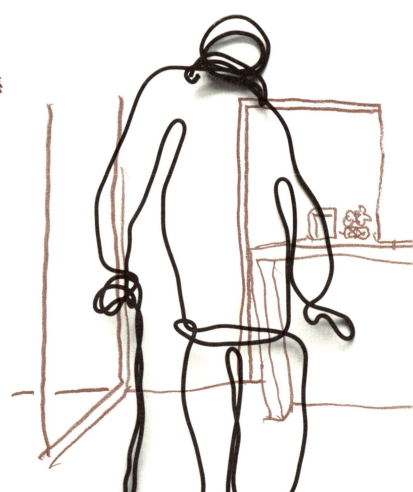

In human care, there's a tendency to fall into a "taking care of" and "being taken care of" relationship.
This makes it impossible to create the kind of positive, open atmosphere I hope to create.
That's why the reception desk at the entrance, which is also the first consultation area,
is built as an open counter — just like all the other counters at all of the facilities.
This spatial arrangement is a sort of prologue to the kind of flat relationships we want to create.
In these areas, the staff carries out not only its reception duties but also its consultation work.
After exchanging greetings and chatting becomes a habit,
the staff will be able to immediately sense changes in guests and be able to initiate conversations.

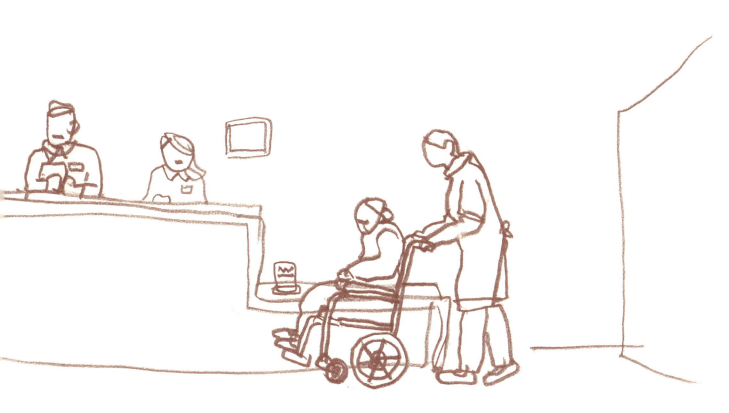

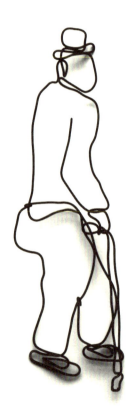

 あえてシロ
Choosing White

私が高齢者施設の計画をスタートした平成4年頃は

今のように施設ごとに個性を競うような時代ではありませんでした。

当時の人々には、「老人ホーム＝暗い、ネガティブ」という形容詞が浮かんでいました。

預ける家族も負い目を感じる人が多かったのです。

そのイメージを払拭するために、空間をカラフルに設える施設もありましたが

幼稚園や小学校のような雰囲気になり、高齢者の尊厳を守れません。

そこで私が考えたのは、真っ白な空間です。

ホワイトカラーは明るく清潔感があり、「はじまりを感じさせる」心理効果があります。

Back in 1992, when I first started designing facilities for the elderly,
we didn't have the kind of competition for originality that we have today.
Back then, people tended to view nursing homes as being dark and depressing.
And families leaving a relative in a home often felt guilty.
To overcome that negative image, some facilities provided colorful spaces.
But that ended up creating an atmosphere like a kindergarten or elementary school,
which damaged the dignity of the elderly residents.
That's why I decided to go with pure white, which has the feeling of brightness and cleanliness.
What's more, it has the psychological effect of a making people feel they're starting something new.

④ むきだしの美
Undressed Beauty

「福祉施設らしからぬ建物」「近代建築との融合」「日本文化を残す」。
龍岡会の建物は、この3つのコンセプトを柱に成しています。
グランドデザインは私の担当。
打ち放しのコンクリートの壁や天井に
木材の窓枠や床がなじむモダンなデザイン。
プリント合板などのフェイク素材は一切使っていません。※
素材の美しさを大切にしたいので、あえてむきだしにこだわりました。

※消防法により定められている箇所を除く

The Tatsuoka Group buildings are designed based on the following three concepts:
(1) they should not look institutional, (2) they are in harmony with modern architecture,
and (3) they preserve a sense of Japanese culture. I'm in charge of the grand design.
I decided on a modern design of undressed concrete walls
and ceilings harmonized with wooden window frames and floors.
The design does not use printed plywood or other man-made
materials unless required legally.*
In order to bring out the natural beauty of the materials,
I deliberately left the materials without alteration.
* Except where prescribed by fire laws.

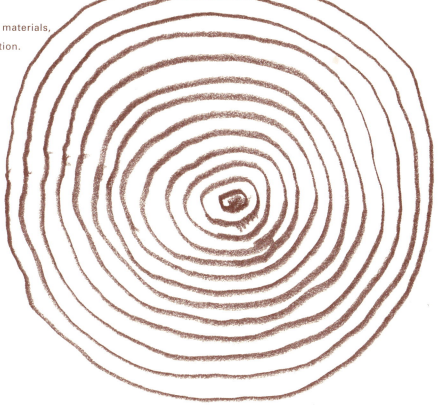

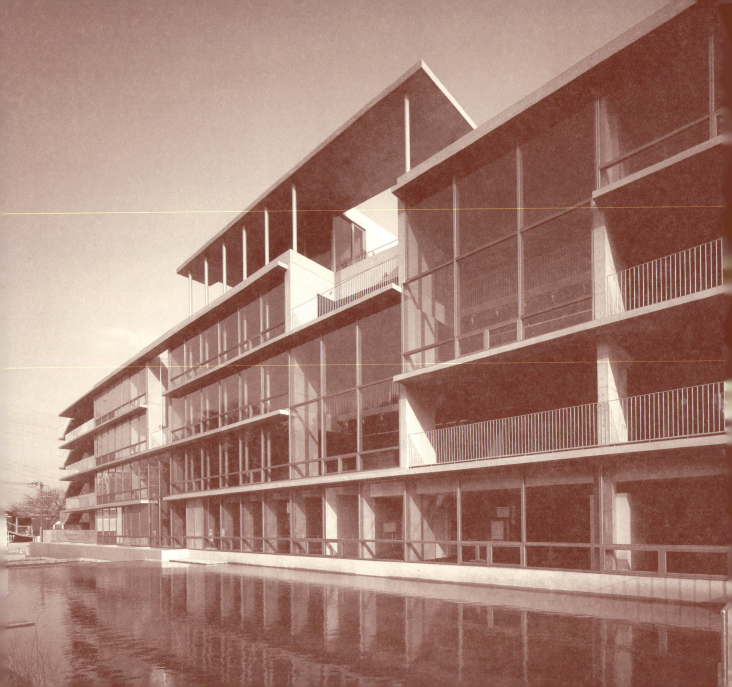

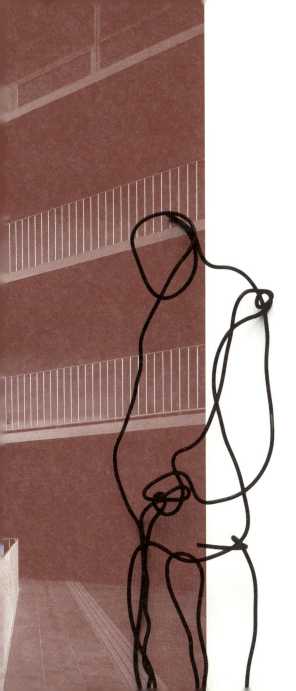

5 門構えからいいものを(ファサード)
High Quality from the Front Gate

『青葉ヒルズ』は2009年にオープンしてから月日が経ちますが
いまだにここを高級マンションだと思っている人が多いようです。
最初から、「門構えから徹底して美しいたたずまい」にこだわりました。
それはひとえに、ゲストの尊厳を守るため。
ゲストには、ここを自分の家として、誇りを持って過ごしてほしい。
ご家族にとっても、訪れるのが楽しみになるような空間にしたかったのです。
おかげさまで『青葉ヒルズ』は、2012年にグッドデザイン賞を受賞しました。

A few years have passed since Aoba Hills opened in 2009, but even today, many people think it's a high-class condominium.
From the beginning, I wanted the building to have an elegant appearance, starting from the front gate.
That's entirely to protect the dignity of the guests.
I want them to think of this as their home and to be proud of living here.
I also want it to be a place that families look forward to visiting.
As a result, Aoba Hills won the 2012 Good Design Award.

壁一面の大きな窓
Wall-sized Windows

大きな窓は、燦々と降り注ぐ陽光や心地よい風の通り道。
自然の恵みを肌で感じると、人は生きるエネルギーを活性化させます。
外出がむずかしいゲストにも季節の風を感じてもらえるよう
どの施設にも天井までつづく大きな窓がたくさんあります。
北側の部屋でも日中は自然光だけで十分なほど。
天候によって明るさが変わるぐらいがちょうどよい。
そんな大らかな気持ちでいられるのも、開放的な窓の効果かもしれません。

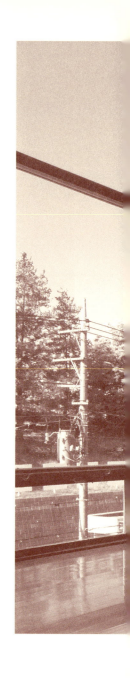

Large windows allow for lots of sunlight and pleasant breezes.
Feeling the blessings of nature on your skin stimulates your energy for living.
That's why all our facilities have large windows stretching all the way
to the ceiling: so that even guests who have a hard time going outside are able to feel the seasons.
With these windows, even the rooms facing north have enough natural light during the day.
How the light changes throughout the day is just about right.
The expansive effect of our windows is most likely what creates this relaxing indoor atmosphere.

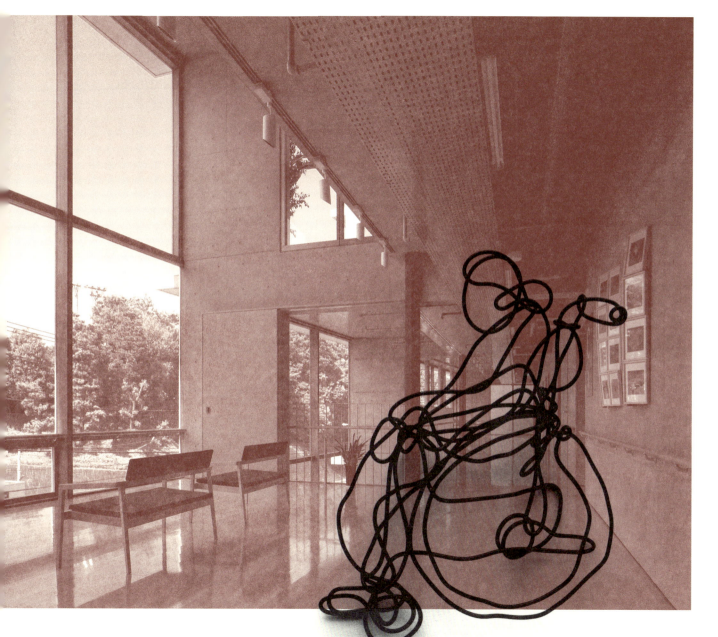

2章 龍岡会を伝える30のキーワード　Chapter 2 30 Key Phrases: The Essence of the Tatsuoka Group

窓から先の風景も考える
Scenery Beyond the Window

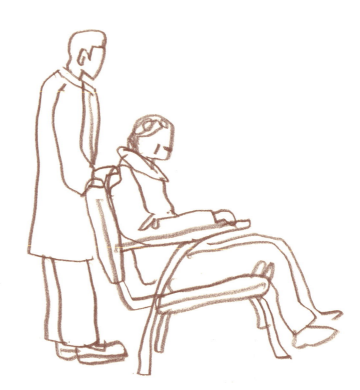

窓からつながる外の景色も、暮らしを彩る大事な要素。
なかなか外に出られないゲストでも、季節を感じることができるような空間を考えます。
たとえば、居室のベッドに横になり、ふと窓に目をやると
四季折々に表情を変える木や花が見えるように、中庭の植栽を計画。
プライベート空間である居室では、心も身体も休めて、静かに過ごしていただきたい。
大きな窓から見える外の景色が、ゲストの心を自然の世界へと誘います。

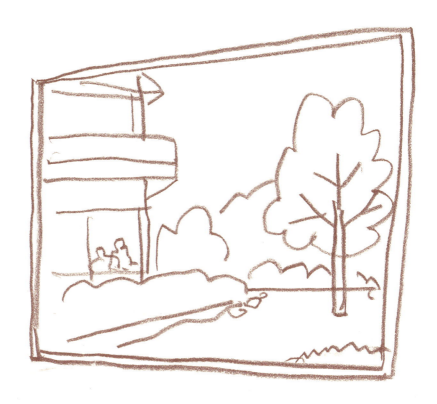

The outside scenery is an important element that lends color to your life.
We tried hard to create a space that would allow guests who can't go outside to feel the seasons too.
For example, we designed the inner courtyard so that if someone lying in bed glances outside,
they'll see trees and flowers that reflect the changing seasons.
When they're in their rooms, they're in their own private space; we want our guests to spend their time peacefully
and to be able to rest their minds and bodies.
The scenery they can see through the large windows will draw their minds into the natural world.

柔らかい光の演出
Soft, Dramatic Light

館内はほとんどが間接照明。
ゲストは仕事や家事に追われることなく
一日の多くを館内でゆっくり過ごすのですから
やすらぎを感じる優しい照明がゲストの暮らしには合います。
大きな窓からは昼は陽光、夜は月光が穏やかに降り注ぐ。
館内はいつでも、柔らかい光のシャワーで包み込まれています。

Most parts of the building have indirect lighting.
Guests spend most of their day inside,
where they don't have to worry about work or chores,
so soft lighting that helps them relax is perfect for their lifestyles.
Sunlight softly streams through the large windows during the day,
and moonlight spills through at night.
The building is continuously bathed in a shower of soft light.

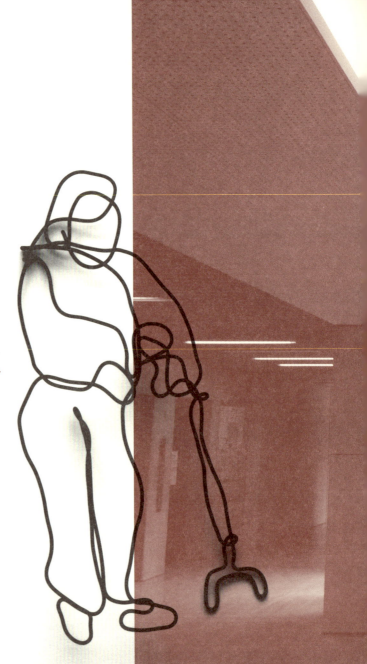

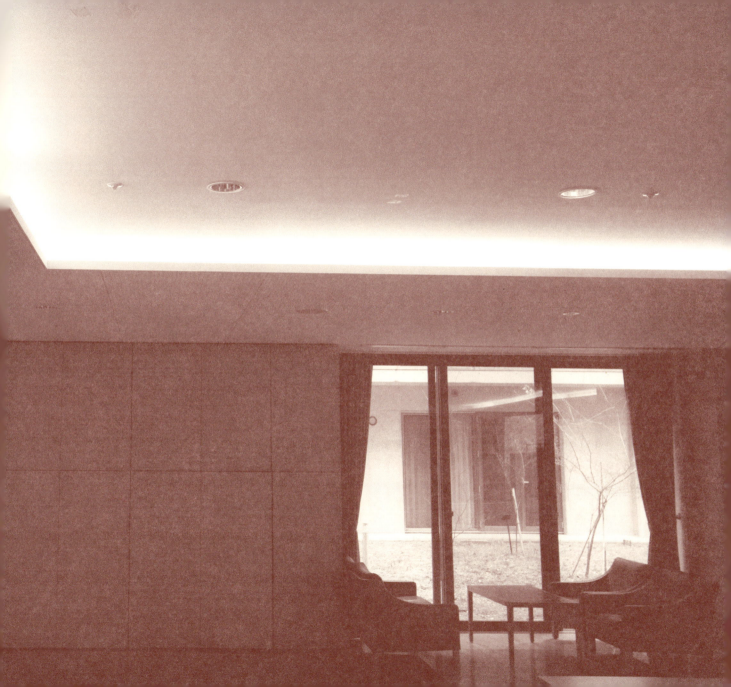

壁に同化するクリーンルーム
Invisible Clean Room

汚物処理室を「Clean Room」と名付けました。
「きれいにしましょう」という意味を込めて
また目立たないように、英語表記のサインにしました。
扉も壁の色に同化させているので、気が付きにくい。
施設はスタッフの職場ではなく、ゲストが生活する空間という意識を大切に。
その他にも、フロアーの冷蔵庫は壁に埋め込み式にするなど
設置する家具や家電も、空間になじむように配慮しています。

The sanitation room is called the "Clean Room."
It's labeled in English because we want to keep the area clean without attracting attention.
The door and wall have similar colors, so the room is difficult to notice.
This is to remind us that this isn't a workplace for our staff; it's a living area for our guests.
Similarly, the refrigerators in the living rooms are embedded in the walls,
and other furniture and household appliances have been installed to match the space they're in, too.

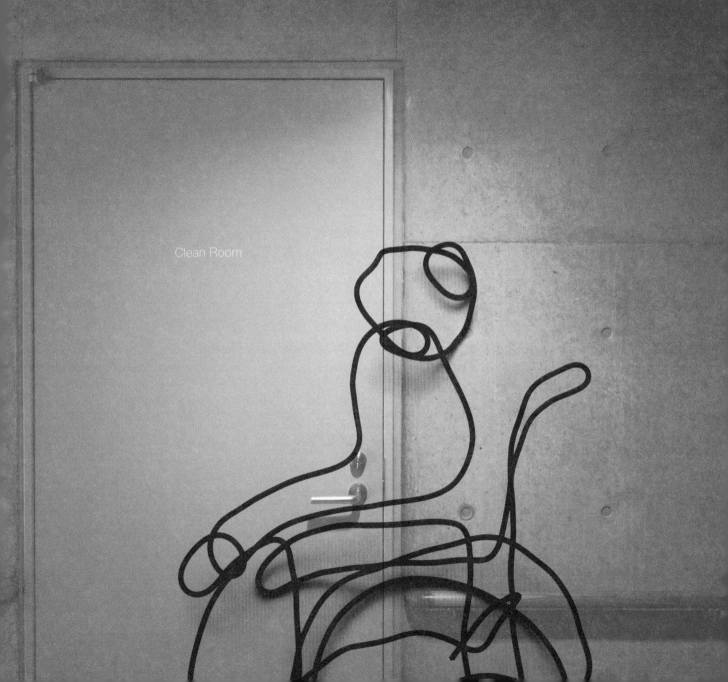

⑩ 一方通行のエレベーター
One-way Elevators

『青葉ヒルズ』のエレベーターは一方通行。
入口と出口が逆にあるので、車椅子の人も向きを変えることなく乗り降りできます。
向きを変えずにすむことで、転倒事故も防げます。
館内で唯一の移動手段となるエレベーターは、閉鎖空間のため匂いがこもったり
ちょっとしたつっかえが事故につながったりすることも。
人・食事・汚物の用途別に使い分けたり、大きな「開閉ボタン」で使いやすくしたり。
人が行き交うコミュニケーションの場でもあるので、ハード面から工夫を凝らしています。

The elevators at Aoba Hills are one-way.
This means that the entrances and exits are on opposite sides,
so people in wheelchairs can get on and off without turning around.
Not having to turn around in the elevators also help to prevent falls and other accidents.
Elevators are the only means of transportation in the building.
Since they're closed spaces, smells can linger, and slight hesitations can lead to accidents.
To improve the situation, separate elevators are used to carry people, meals, and waste.
And to make the elevators easier to use, a large open-close button has been installed.
Elevators are places of communication where residents often meet,
so we've put a lot of ingenuity into improving them.

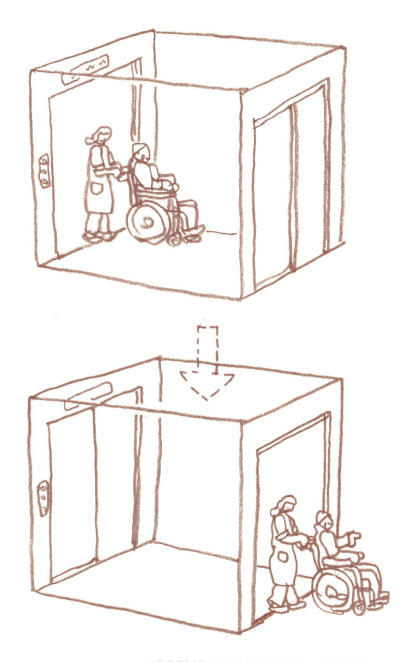

押しても引いても開くドア
Our Special Doors

トイレは入るときにドアを「押す」、出るときにも「押す」。
これは、押しても引いても開くドアだからこそできる技。
「引く」動作でバランスを崩し後ろに転倒する、そんな事故も防ぎます。
高齢になるとトイレの回数が増えて、夜中に寝ぼけ眼でトイレへ行くことも。
ちょっとした工夫で暮らしの安全性はグンと高まります。
だから、設えからすべてをオーダーメイドにしています。

To enter the bathroom, you push; to leave, you push.
The special door provides safety.
Pulling can cause people to lose balance and fall backwards, but these doors prevent such accidents.
Older people go to the bathroom more often, and sometimes they go at night while they're half asleep.
This clever design makes their lives a whole lot safer.
That's why all our doors were customized from the very beginning.

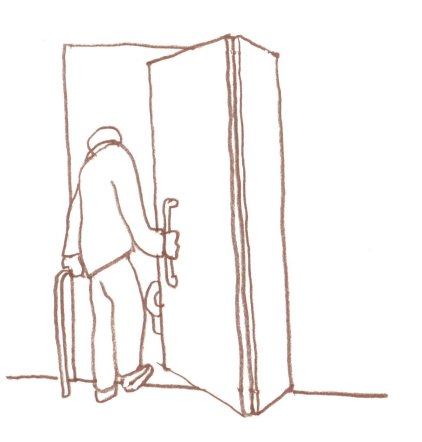
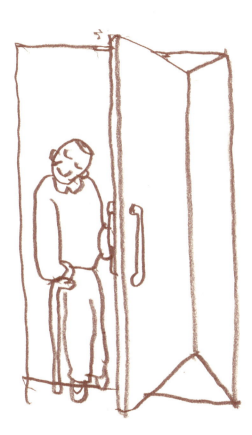

2章 龍岡会を伝える30のキーワード　　Chapter 2　30 Key Phrases: The Essence of the Tatsuoka Group

長生きする素材
Long-living Materials

日本は木の文化。
それは、火山によって土壌が豊かになり、四季もあり
雨がよく降るので、木が育ちやすいからだといわれています。
木は長く使えば使うほど、風合いが出る。
そして木は、人が長生きできる素材でもあるのです。
ある大学の研究で、マウスを木・コンクリート・鉄骨の3つの檻で過ごさせたところ
木の檻のマウスが、一番長生きしたという結果が出たそうです。
これは、私ができる限り内装に木を使っている理由のひとつです。

Japan's culture is a "culture of wood."
This is because volcanoes have made the soil fertile,
and with frequent rainfall and four seasons, trees grow easily.
The longer you use wood, the more the texture appears.
Wood is also a material that helps people to live longer.
In one university study, mice were raised in separate cages made of wood, concrete, and steel.
The researchers discovered that the mice in the wooden cage lived the longest.
This connection to longevity is one reason why I use wood for the interior as much as possible.

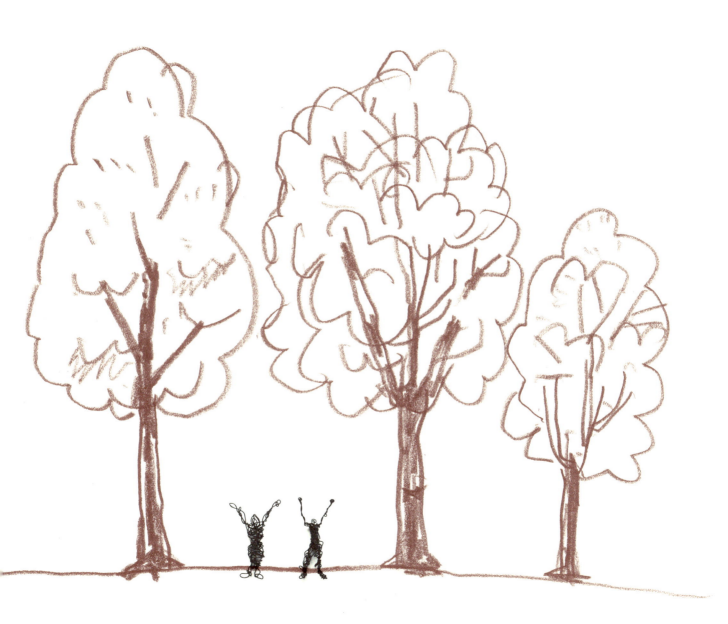

⑬ ウッドデッキで BBQ
Barbecue Parties

ウッドデッキでのBBQは龍岡会の夏の風物詩。
みんなで育てた、採れたての野菜で肉を巻き、青空の下で大宴会。
見晴らしがよく心地よい風に、解放感も抜群です。
たとえば『櫻川』『千壽』では、花火大会を眺めることもできます。
ウッドデッキやバルコニーは、避難経路のひとつです。
いざというときにどの方向にも避難できるように、車椅子が通れる幅を十分に確保。
建物をぐるりと囲むように取り付けています。

Barbecue parties out on the wooden deck are a Tatsuoka Group summer tradition.
Eating meat wrapped in vegetables they've raised and just harvested,
the guests, family members, and staff all enjoy a banquet under the blue sky together.
The beautiful views and comfortable breezes bring an unrivaled sense of liberation.
For example, at our Sakuragawa and Senju facilities, guests can also enjoy fireworks displays.
The wooden decks and balconies also serve as evacuation routes.
They are fully secured with outdoor passages wide enough for wheelchairs,
so that in the case of an emergency, guests can evacuate in any direction.
Such decks and balconies are attached to all sides of the building.

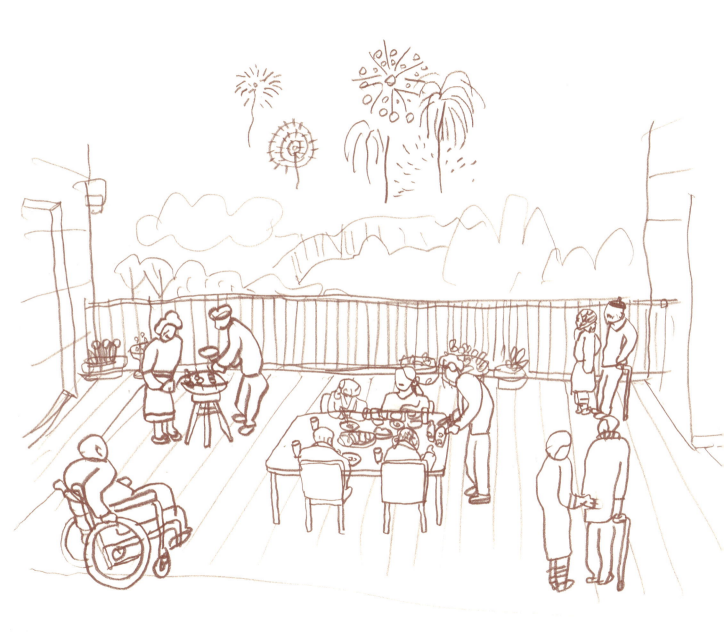

2章 龍岡会を伝える30のキーワード　　Chapter 2 30 Key Phrases: The Essence of the Tatsuoka Group

14 静の空間、動の空間
Stillness and Motion

高齢になると、環境に順応することがむずかしくなってきます。
だから介護施設では、設計の段階から
"ソフトに基づいたハード"を綿密に考えることが大切。
私が考えたコンセプトは、メリハリのある空間です。

When you get older, it becomes increasingly difficult to adapt to the environment.
For this reason, human care facilities need to thoroughly consider
the human dimensions even from the planning stage.
One concept I considered was to have customized spaces for different purposes.

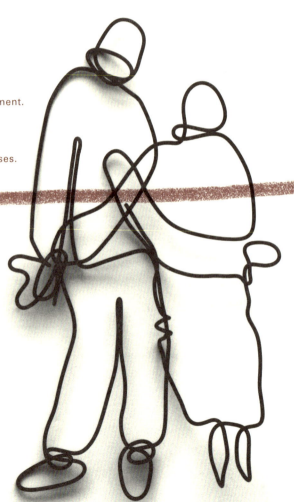

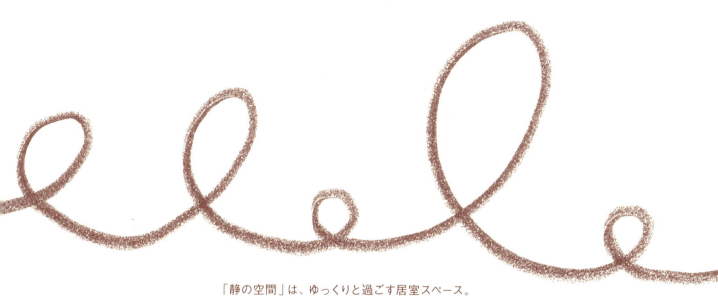

「静の空間」は、ゆっくりと過ごす居室スペース。
自然に囲まれて、静かに内観する時間が流れます。
一方で「動の空間」は、レクリエーションやリハビリを行う共用部。
人が行き交い、暮らしにアクセントを与えます。
館内に居ながらにして、空間ごとに世界が変わるような動線を考えました。

Private living areas spent relaxing are spaces of stillness for relaxation.
In these areas, people are surrounded by nature, and spend their time in calm introspection.
Common areas used for recreation and rehabilitation, on the other hand, are spaces of motion.
In these areas, people come and go, and energy is added to their lives.
I came up with flow lines that allow the world to completely change
as you enter different spaces—even while remaining in the same building.

近すぎず、遠すぎず
Not Too Close, Not Too Far

介護をする人とされる人の距離感は、"近すぎず、遠すぎず"くらいが丁度よい。
家族ではなく、家族のようなスタッフだからこそ
思いやりを持った関係が築きやすい面もあります。
そんな距離感を、空間づくりにも反映しています。
モダンな吹き抜けのある施設でも、居室の天井は低めに設定。
『青葉ヒルズ』のショートステイエリアは
中庭をはさんでお互いの暮らしが感じられる、向き合わせのユニットです。

The perfect sense of distance between those giving and those receiving care is
one that's not too close but not too far away.
Staff members aren't family but they are almost like family,
and different kind of interactions help to foster friendly relations.
This sense of distance is also reflected in how spaces in the building have been created.
For example, even in facilities with a modern-style high-ceilinged atrium,
the ceiling in the private quarters are much lower.
The short-term resident area at Aoba Hills has units that are
facing one another from opposite sides of the courtyard, to allow for a sense of community.

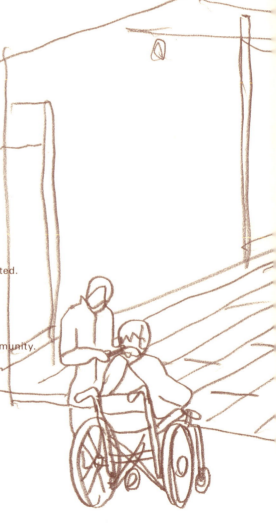

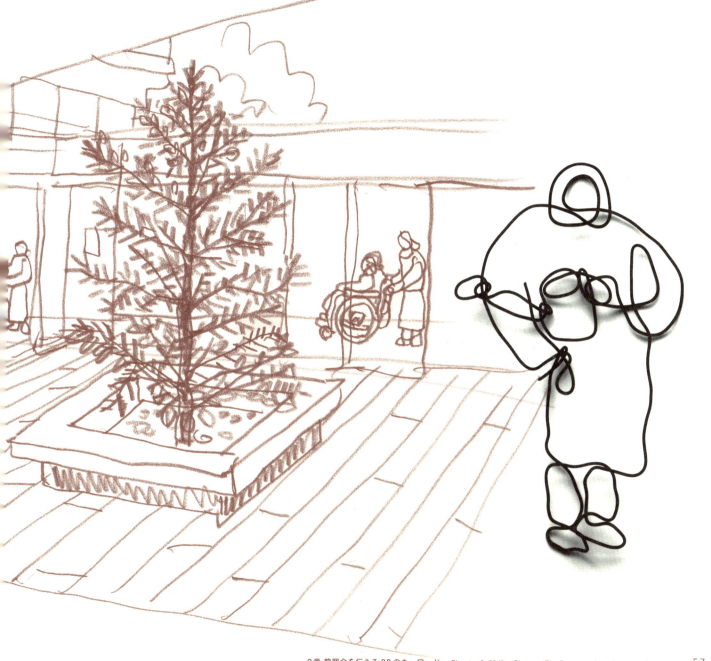

16 北欧家具のシークレット
The Magic of Scandinavian Furniture

龍岡会の家具はすべて北欧製。椅子、ソファ、テーブル、ベッドまで
日本人が合うサイズにセミオーダーしています。
北欧製の椅子は長時間座ってもまったく苦にならず、座り心地が抜群。
椅子の文化が浅い日本にはかなわない"シークレット技術"が
北欧にはあるのでは？と、思わずにはいられません。
昔から、福祉先進国を謳う北欧では、高温で洗えるファブリック製の椅子が主流です。
対して日本の施設は「失禁してもすぐに拭き取れる方がよい」という発想でビニール製。
どちらの方が使い心地がよいのかは……明白ですよね。

The Tatsuoka Group always uses Scandinavian furniture.
Our chairs, sofas, tables, and even our beds are semi-customized to Japanese sizes.
Scandinavian chairs are very comfortable; you can sit on them for hours without any stress.
I can't help thinking there are some secret techniques that Japan,
which is still relatively inexperienced with the chair culture, can't possibly figure out.
In Scandinavia, where they advocate the virtues of the advanced welfare state,
chairs made with fabric that can be washed at high temperatures have long been the norm.
Japanese facilities, however, have usually opted for plastic,
based on the idea that in the event of incontinence, they can immediately be wiped clean.
So which type of chair is more comfortable? Of course, the answer is obvious.

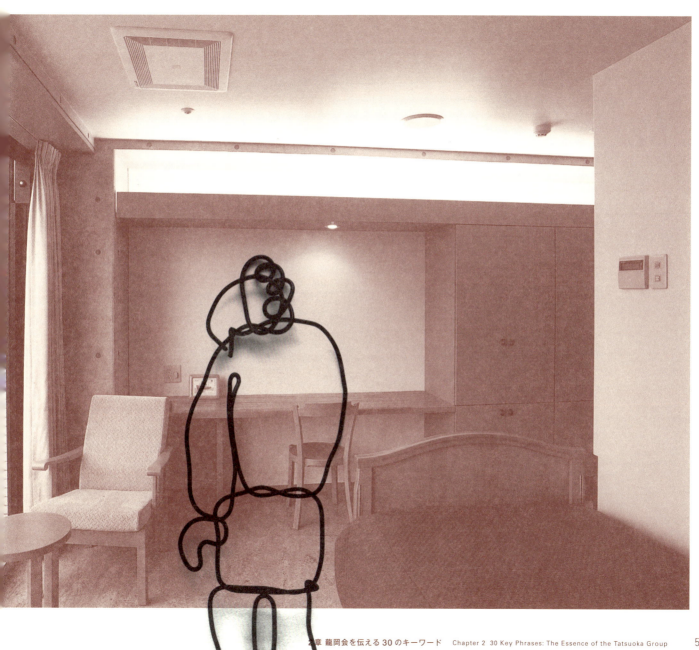

2章 龍岡会を伝える30のキーワード　　Chapter 2 30 Key Phrases: The Essence of the Tatsuoka Group

⑰ どこにでも椅子
Chairs Everywhere

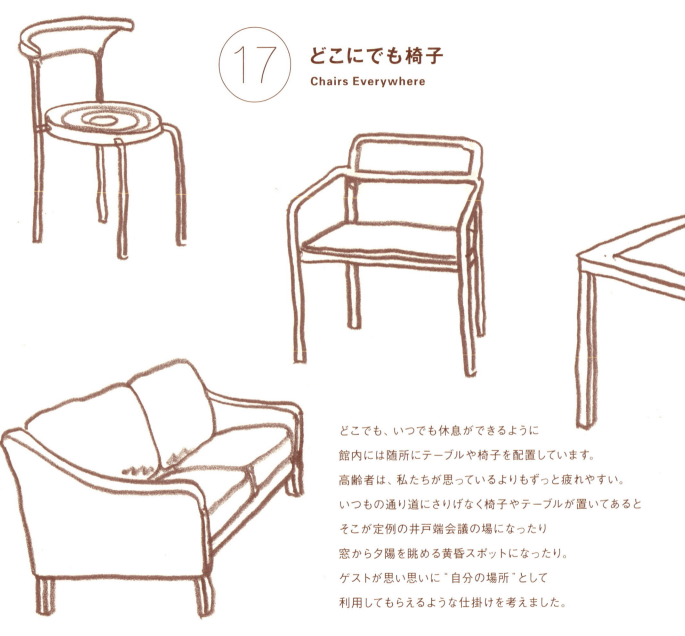

どこでも、いつでも休息ができるように
館内には随所にテーブルや椅子を配置しています。
高齢者は、私たちが思っているよりもずっと疲れやすい。
いつもの通り道にさりげなく椅子やテーブルが置いてあると
そこが定例の井戸端会議の場になったり
窓から夕陽を眺める黄昏スポットになったり。
ゲストが思い思いに"自分の場所"として
利用してもらえるような仕掛けを考えました。

Tables and chairs are located throughout the building so that guests can rest anytime and anywhere.
Older people get fatigued much more easily than you think.
If chairs and tables have been unobtrusively placed along the regular routes,
they naturally become places for coffee klatches, watching the sunset, or other pleasant habits.
This was a clever way to let our guests find their own special spots on their own.

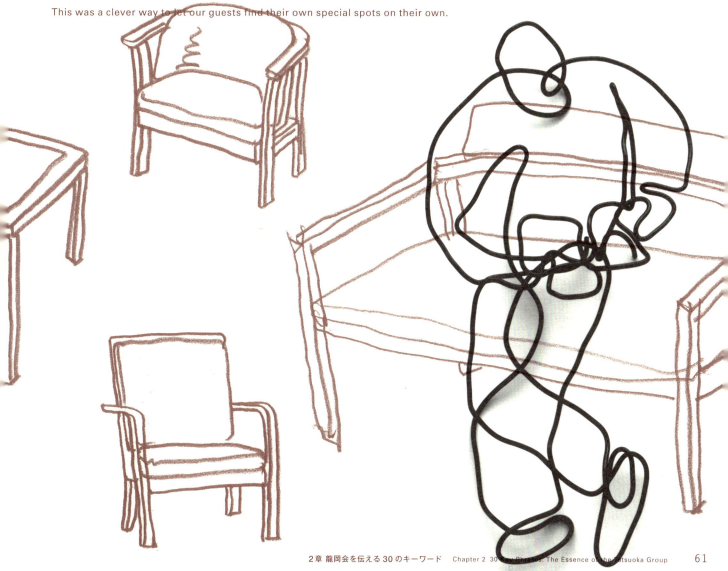

子どもあつかいしないサイン
Signs That are Simple, Not Childish

看板やロゴなどのサインは、白内障や緑内障の人でも情報がきちんと伝わるように
壁の色と相性がよい色をカラーユニバーサルデザインから選びました。
サインには、著名なグラフィックデザイナーの
洗練されたデザインを採用しています。
どこでも、誰にとっても、わかりやすく、センスよく。
毎日目にするものだからこそ、美しいものにこだわります。

For signboards, logos, and other signs,
I chose pleasant colors from Color Universal Design or Colorblind Barrier Free
that match the color of the wall and that can effectively convey information
to people with cataracts or glaucoma.
For the designs, I chose elegant ones created by well-known graphic designers.
Anyone anywhere would consider them to be tasteful and easy to understand.
Signs are things we look at every day, so I really wanted them to be attractive.

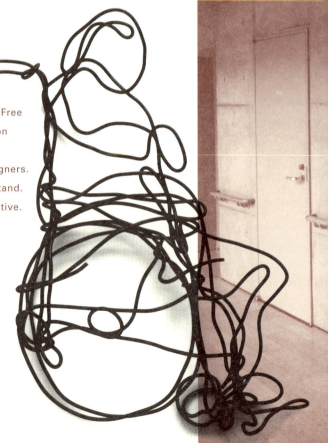

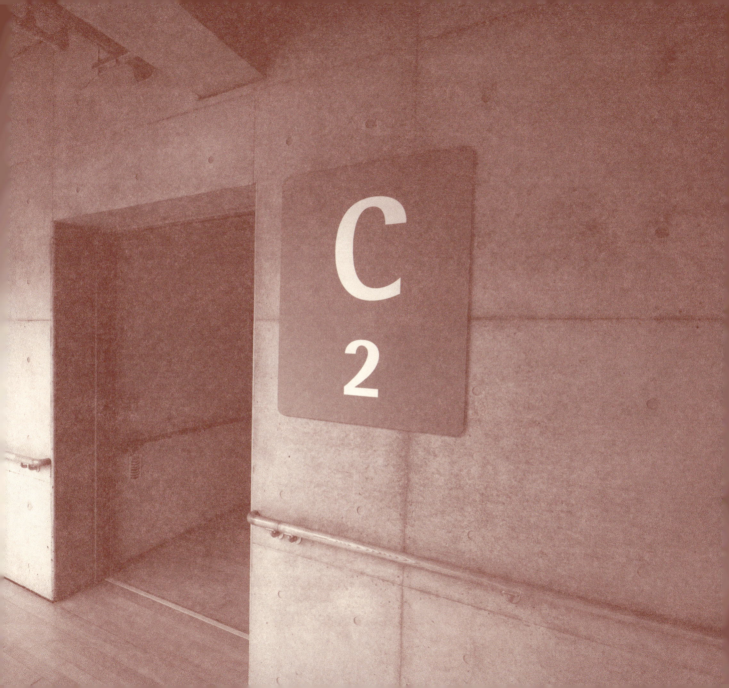

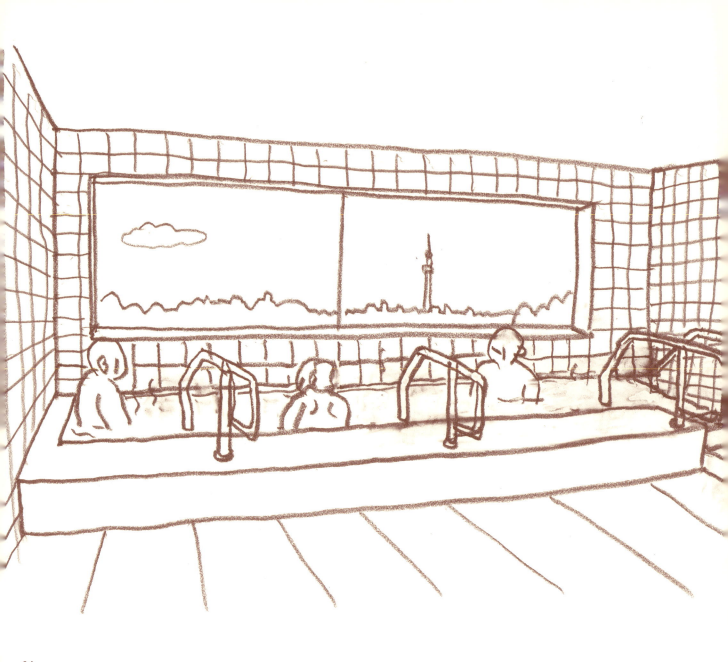

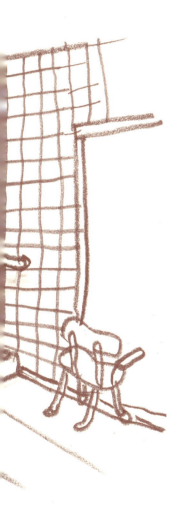

湯船に浸かるのはニッポンの文化
Soaking in the Bath: It's Part of Being Japanese

龍岡会の入浴設備は、寝たまま浸かるような機械浴はほとんどありません。
代わりに、大浴場に座ったままで入れるリフトを設置しています。
「あぁ、いい湯だな〜」と湯船に浸かるのが、日本人ならではの至福のひととき。
大きな湯船にみんなで浸かると、話も弾むものです。
入浴ケアーは事故のリスクが高く、細心の注意を払いますが
一度に入る人数を決めたり、スタッフの人数を増やしたりして
ゲストが満足ゆくまで、お風呂を楽しんでいただけるように努めています。

The Tatsuoka Group doesn't have many individual mechanical baths that
put you in the bath in a reclining position.
Instead, we've installed lifts that put you in the large communal bath in a sitting position.
For most Japanese, soaking in the bath and enjoying the warm water is a time of supreme bliss.
When everyone is soaking in a large bath together, the conversation becomes lively.
Since bathing has a high risk of accidents, we take scrupulous care to avoid problems by
limiting the number of people that enter at one time and by increasing the number of staff.
We do our best to help our guests enjoy their bath time.

おいしさは脳で感じる
Umami is in the Mind

今は、科学が進化して「うま味」成分が発見されたりする時代。
でも私は、本当のおいしさは脳で感じるものだと思っています。
だから、ご飯とお味噌汁は、ユニットごとのキッチンで毎食スタッフがつくっています。
ご飯とお味噌汁は、家族の食卓の象徴です。
また、嗅覚の刺激は本能に直結するといわれています。
食事時間が近づくと、湯気や香りがフロアー内に漂い
認知症の方も「ご飯かな?」と、ひょっこり顔をのぞかせます。

Recently, science has evolved to discover *umami* as a component.
But I think people really sense deliciousness in their minds.
That's why our staff makes rice and miso soup for every meal, right there in each unit's kitchen.
In Japan, rice and miso soup symbolize the family dining table.
And since it is said that olfactory stimulation is directly connected to instinct,
we want the steam and smells to float out across the floor,
so that even someone with dementia will suddenly perk up and notice that it's mealtime.

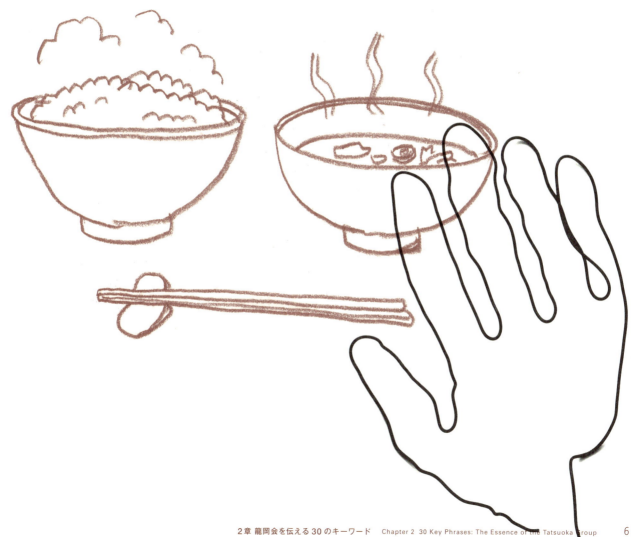

食の30秒ルール
The 30-second Rule for Hot Meals

「温かいものは温かく、冷たいものは冷たく」。
暮らしの中で一番の楽しみともいえる食事への配慮は、スタッフ総出で取り組みます。
目標は、盛り付けてから30秒以内に、ゲストの口に入ること。
毎食、ゲストが席についてから盛りつけるので
できたてホカホカの食事が提供できています。
大人数の食事を一気に用意するのは大変な労力ですが
ゲストの立場に立って考えると、当たり前のことなのです。

We believe that warm food should be served warm, and cold food should be served cold.
Mealtime, which is often the greatest pleasure of a person's day, is a priority for our entire staff.
Our goal is to allow guests to start eating within 30 seconds after the food is served.
Every meal is served after our guests are seated, so we can serve hot, freshly cooked food.
A lot of work goes into preparing meals for a large group of people,
but when we consider our guests, we feel this is the least we can do.

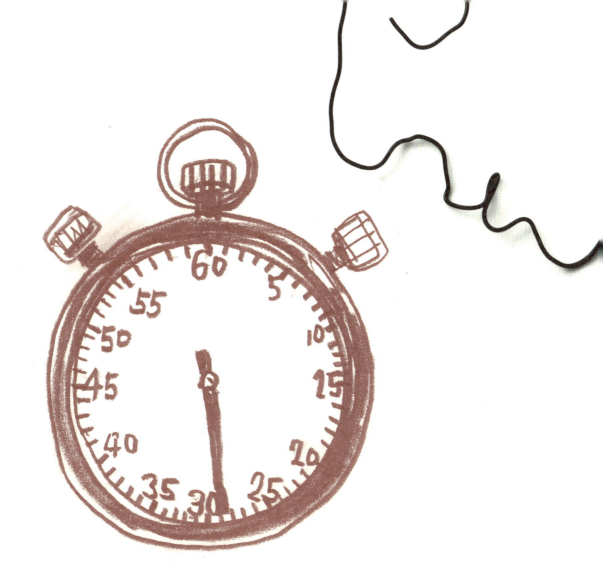

好きなものを、みんなで一緒に
Sharing the Joys of Favorite Foods Together

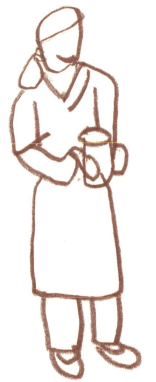

たとえば病院では、事前に食事メニューを渡して
あらかじめ食べるものを決めてもらうことが多い。
龍岡会では、昼夜の食事とおやつは、その日そのときの気分で選んでいただきます。
これは、食材の仕入れや調理のことを考えると、なかなかむずかしい。
そこで私は、スタッフもゲストと同じ食事を、同じテーブルでとるようにしました。
ゲストがどんな食事を食べているのかは、実際に食べてみるのが一番。
賑やかな食卓になるだけではなく、メニューのアイデアも生まれる、一石二鳥の名案です。

At hospitals, for example, we often hand our guests a menu and
let them chose what they'll eat in advance.
At our facilities, we let our guests choose their afternoon snacks and morning and
evening meals based on how they're feeling that very day.
When you consider the difficulties of cooking and stocking food, you'll realize this is no small task.
To foster understanding, I decided that staff and guests should eat the same food at the same tables.
This is really the best way to understand what our guests are eating.
Not only does this make for lively meals, but it also gives us new ideas for the menu.
It's a nice policy that kills two birds with one stone.

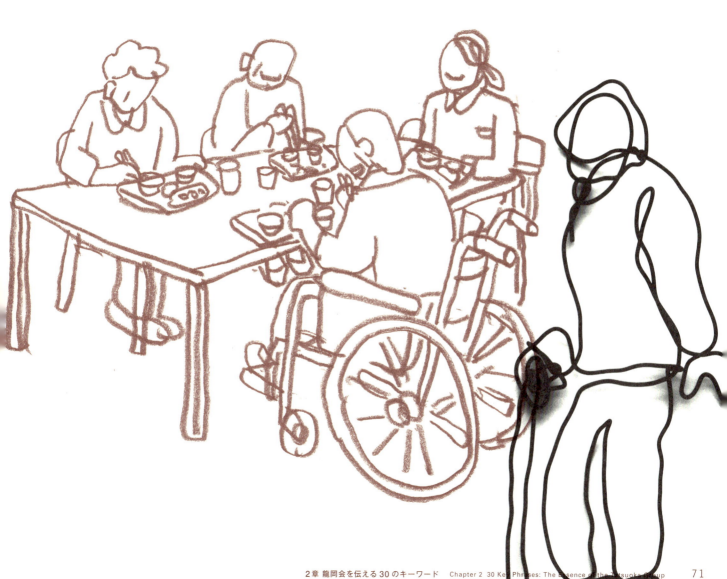

㉓ 介護食のイノベーション
Innovative Human-care Food

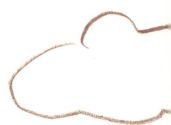
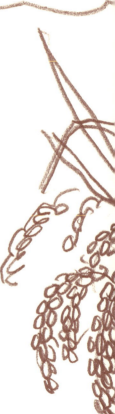

龍岡会では2012年より、介護食改革をスタート。

醤油、酒、味噌などの基本調味料を、無添加のものに切り替えました。

また、新潟県南魚沼郡湯沢町の休耕地を借りて、無農薬の米作りにも挑戦。

実はこれは、食育も兼ねています。

スタッフの子どもも参加して、稲作に励みました。

他にも、リンゴは長野県へ収穫に行きます。

食の安全と美味しさへの探究心、それが、ゲストが満足できる食事につながると考えています。

In 2012, the Tatsuoka Group initiated a reform of its food policy.

To begin with, we switched to using additive-free basic seasonings, such as soy sauce, sake (rice wine), and miso.

More ambitiously, we borrowed a piece of fallow land from the town of
Yuzawa in the Minami-Uonuma District of Niigata Prefecture and started raising our own pesticide-free rice.

The project has an educational component as well.

Children of staff members have also participated in working hard to grow rice.

In addition, we go to Nagano Prefecture to pick apples.

I believe this spirit of inquiry concerning food safety and
taste helps us provide satisfying meals to our guests.

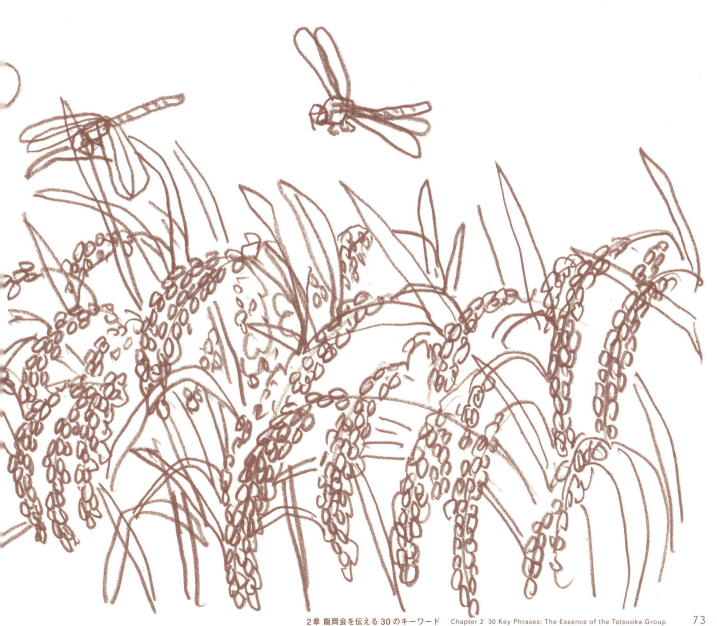

24 ハーティーミール®
Hearty Meal®

「ハーティーミール®」は私たちがつくった言葉で、"心のこもった食事"という意味。

「食べる意欲が命を再生させる」と信じています。

だから龍岡会では、ゲストが最期に食べたいものを食べられるようにつくる

という課題に、チャレンジし続けています。

メニューは鰻だったり、お煎餅だったり……。やっぱりみなさん、日本食が多いですね。

どんなに身体の状態が悪くても、顔をほころばせて、美味しそうに召し上がります。

※Hearty Meal® は、特許庁で登録されている登録商標です

Hearty Meal® is a phrase we came up with to refer to meals that are made from the heart.
I believe a healthy appetite restores life.
That's why we remain committed to providing the meals that our guests want to eat during their final years.
Sometimes they want eel; sometimes, rice crackers. Not surprisingly, most of our guests like Japanese food.
We're pleased to see that even those in poor physical condition always eat with a smile on their face.
*Hearty Meal® is a trademark registered in the Japan Patent Office (JPO).

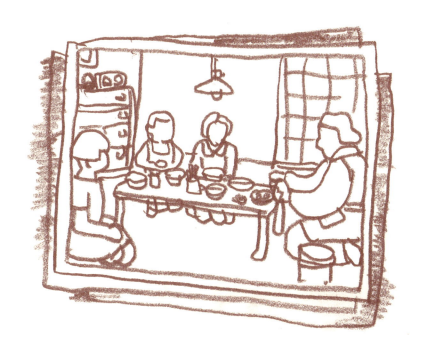

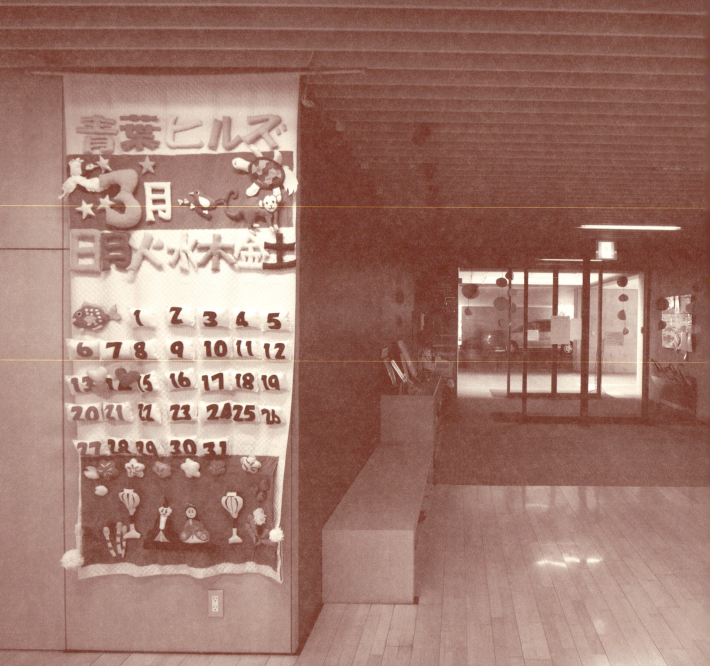

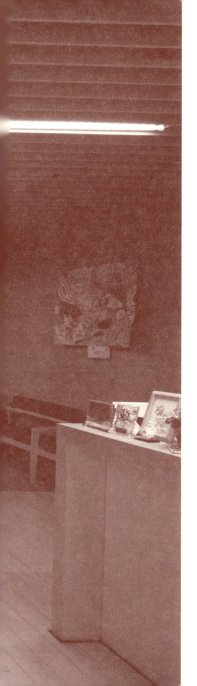

25 スタッフは芸術家
Staff Who are Artists

「人生にアートは欠かせない」。
これは私の生き方の美学。アートは生活に彩りをもたらしてくれます。
また、音楽や絵を描くことは、医学的にリハビリ効果も期待できるのです。
そして、何でも本物を取り入れるのが龍岡会の方針。
美大や音大を卒業したスタッフを迎えて、ゲストと一緒に作品づくりを行っています。
プロが導くと、ゲストの作品の完成度もずいぶん上がります。
1998年にはホテルオークラで、2011年には帝国ホテルで展覧会を開催しました。

I believe that art is an indispensable part of life.
In fact, this is my philosophy of living. Art brings color and spice into our daily lives.
In addition, music and drawing pictures has been medically shown to
have a rehabilitating effect on people.
Since the Tatsuoka Group's policy has always been to incorporate genuine articles,
we invite staff members who have graduated from art and
music colleges to create artistic works with our guests.
With professionals leading the way,
our guests have raised the quality of their works to even higher levels.
In 1998, we held an exhibition at Hotel Okura; in 2011, at the Imperial Hotel.

26 ケアーサイエンス®＝答えを出す
Care Science® = Finding Answers

「Evidence Based Medicine（根拠に基づいた医療）」という言葉を基に
「Care Science®」「Evidence Based Care®」という言葉をつくりました。
データに基づいた最適なケアーを提供することは
医療では当然のことでも、介護では実現できていないのが現状です。
たとえば、認知症の方の問題行動には必ず理由がある。
でも彼らは自分で意思を伝えることができないので、臨床データが必要です。
龍岡会では日頃からデータを収集し
国際学会にも積極的にエントリーするようにしています。

※ケアーサイエンス®、Care Science®、Evidence Based Care®は、特許庁で登録されている登録商標です

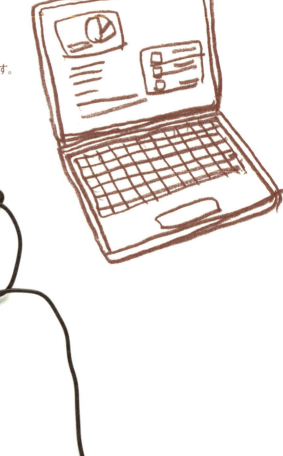

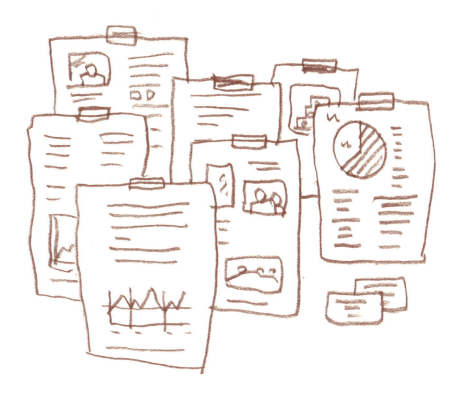

Care Science® and Evidence Based Care® are concepts we came up with
in order to expand evidence-based medicine to the field of human care.
Providing appropriate care based on data is routine in hospitals, but human care is currently lagging behind.
For example, there's certainly a reason why people with dementia behave the way they do.
However, they can't convey their desires, so clinical data is needed.
To find answers, the Tatsuoka Group has been collecting data regularly and
making positive contributions to international research societies.
*Care Science® and Evidence Based Care® are trademarks registered in the Japan Patent Office (JPO).

27 小さな夢を叶えるプロジェクト
Making Modest Dreams Come True

龍岡会では、「もう一度行きたい場所へ行く」リクエストを受け付け中。
ゲストが希望する先は、新婚旅行で訪れた場所や
幼少時代に通っていた小学校など、思い出の場所が多いです。
もちろん計画段階から、医師や看護師、ケアースタッフがチームを組んで
健康面・安全面の配慮も万全に整えます。
その日を励みに元気になっていくゲストの姿を見るのが、何よりうれしい。
ゲストのささやかな夢を共に達成する喜びは、格別です。

The Tatsuoka Group accepts requests from guests for places they'd like to revisit.
Requests have included places visited during honeymoons,
elementary schools attended when they were young, and other places connected to fond memories.
From the planning stage, of course, our doctors, nurses, and staff work together as a team so that all measures are
taken to ensure the health and safety of participants.
It makes us so happy to see how encouraged and cheerful our guests become for these trips.
Sharing the joy of guests as their modest dreams come true is indeed a special experience.

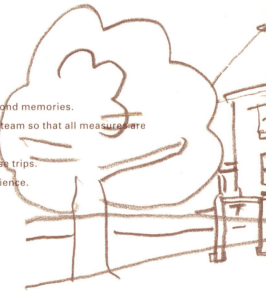

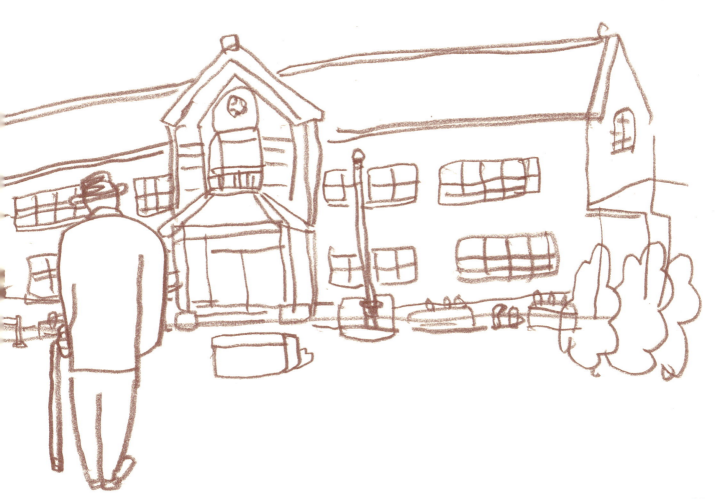

㉘ 外出のもうひとつの狙い
The Other Goal of Outings

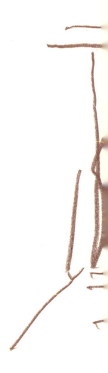

外出イベントは、映画鑑賞や国技館での相撲鑑賞、温泉など、どこへでも積極的に出かけます。
一番の目的は、ゲストのリフレッシュや社会参加のため。
もうひとつは、外へ働きかけることで
社会整備を高齢者に寄り添ったものに変えていって欲しい、という思いがあります。
以前は、映画館の車椅子スペースが一番前に設置されていたり
高速SAの福祉車の駐車場が、トイレから離れた場所にあったりしました。
その都度、私たちは、施設へ意見を伝えるなど、アクションを起こしてきました。

We're extremely positive about taking our guests on outings to the movies,
sumo tournaments, hot springs, and various events.
The main goal is for our guests to enjoy themselves and feel like members of society.
But another goal is to influence the outside world,
so that public facilities and services become friendlier to the elderly.
Previously, movie theaters put spaces for wheelchairs all the way at the front,
and highway service areas had their handicapped parking spots far from the bathrooms.
When we've encountered such problems, we've contacted the concerned establishment or
taken other action to facilitate change.

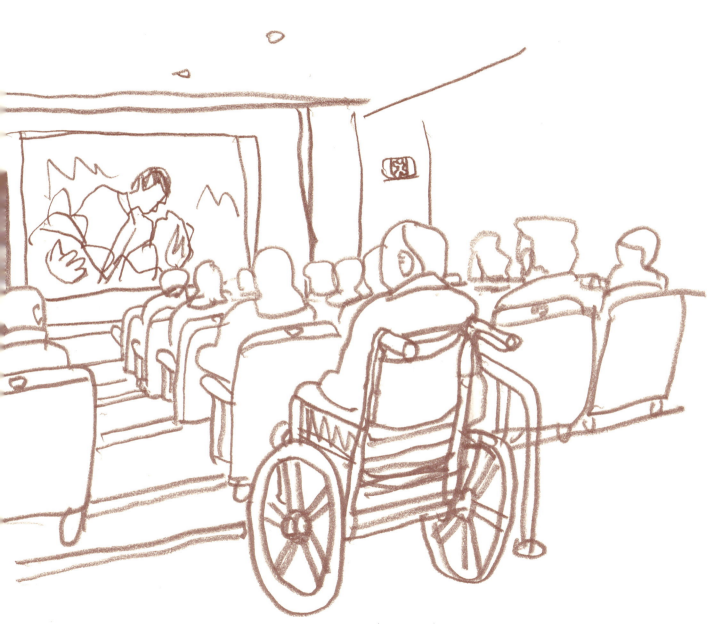

地域への架け橋
Bridges to the Local Community

『龍岡会』は「龍岡」、『青葉ヒルズ』は「青葉台」、『千壽』は「千住」など
実は施設名は、そこの地名をもじっています。
地域に対する愛情や敬意は、できるだけ形で表わしたいと考えています。
例えば『千壽』が建っている土地は、元は染め工場。
だから、浴室の暖簾は千住の街並みを描いた染め物に
壁面や天井の塗装には、わずかに藍の塗料を混ぜました。
その思いが、地域との架け橋になっています。

Our facilities have names that invoke the historical names.
In as many ways as possible, we want to express our love and respect for the local communities.
For example, our Senju facility is located where there used to be a dye factory,
so the entrance to the facility's bathing area has dividing curtains of dyed cloth
with images of the Senju cityscape, and the walls and ceilings are painted
with paint that has some indigo-dyed paint mixed in.
This positive attitude helps us to be a bridge to the local community.

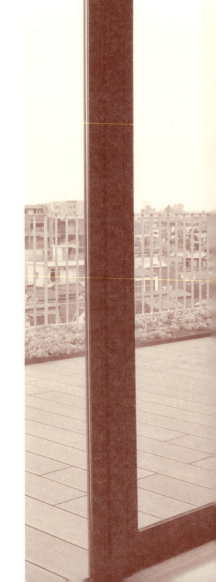

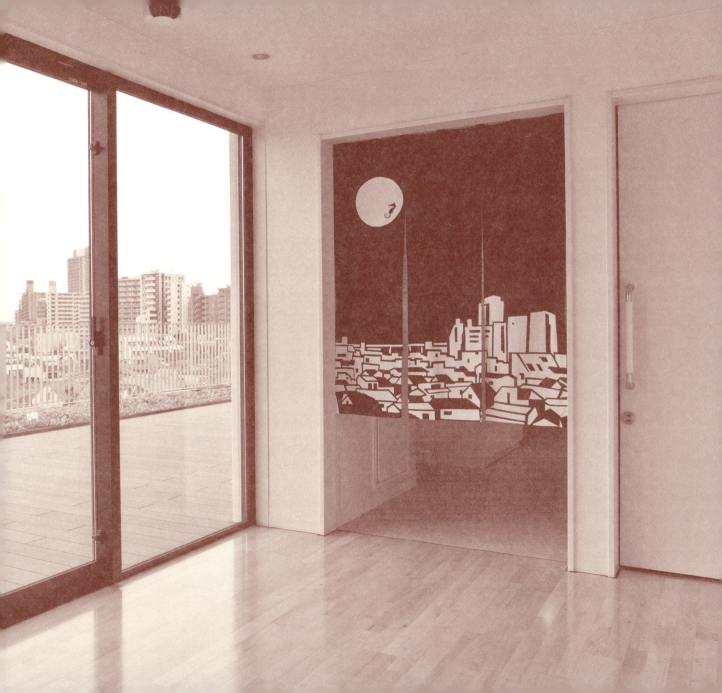

㉚ 介護に国境はない
No Borders in Human Care

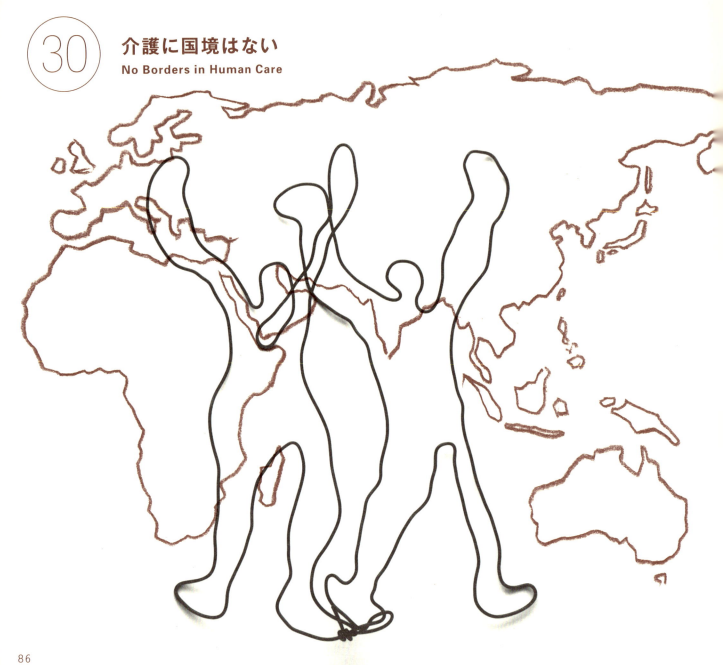

長生きすることは、人類誰もが望むこと。
とはいえ、先進国のどの国でも、高齢化問題への対応は急務。
老いは、人種や宗教に関係なく、景気の流れにも無関係。とどまることがありません。
国境を越えて、みんなで学び考えていくことが、明るい未来をつくるのです。
そんな思いから、龍岡会では、海外からの視察を積極的に受け入れています。
また、スタッフには年に一度、北欧をはじめとした海外研修を実施。
世界の文化を肌で感じ、見聞を広めて欲しいと思っています。
スタッフの人生が豊かになると、結果としていいケアーにつながるからです。

All human beings want to live for a long time.
Even so, many advanced nations still need to get serious about dealing with their aging populations.
Growing old is something all of us must confront, regardless of race, religion, or economic background.
There's no stopping it. Only by learning from one another, without regard to national borders, can we can build a bright future.
With this in mind, the Tatsuoka Group warmly welcomes overseas visitors to tour our facilities.
At the same time, we provide our staff with yearly overseas training in Denmark, Sweden, Norway, Finland, England, Germany, Holland, France, Australia and other areas.
We want them to directly experience the cultures of the world and to expand their store of knowledge.
If their lives are enriched, the care they provide will improve, too.

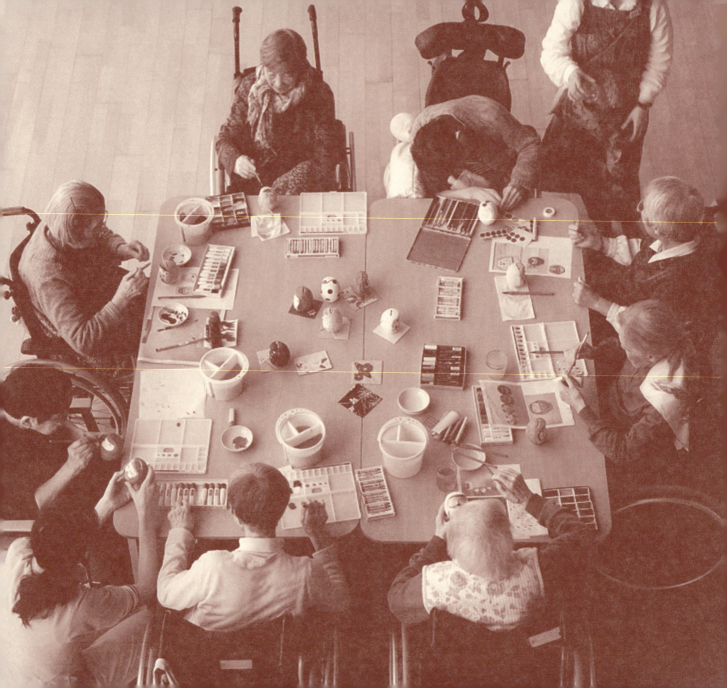

3章 インタビュー スタッフの取り組み
Chapter 3 Interviews: Staff Endeavor

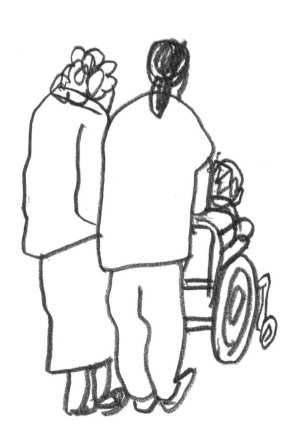

介護部の取り組み
一生青春、一生感動

「サッカー選手になりたかった」という『青葉ヒルズ』のケアースタッフ・星英介さん。夢を追いかけて、Jリーグの試験をチャレンジし続けていく中で、生活のために入った介護の世界。気がつけば、介護歴約15年。今では、フロアー主任としてスタッフを束ねる存在だ。そんな星さんが関わってきたプロジェクトのひとつに、「もういちど行きたい場所へ行く」という外出企画がある。

「2年前に、"日本一大きな花火を見たい"というゲストがいたときは、新潟県の長岡花火大会へ、日帰り弾丸ツアーを決行。僕の故郷だったので、運転手役からツアー企画まで、中心になって考えました。まずは、信州そばや塩沢産コシヒカリのおむすびなど、旅の途中でその土地ならではのものを食べられるお店のリストアップから。旅は目的地へ行くまでの小さな思い出が記憶に残るものなので、コースはシミュレーションしながら綿密に考えました」。

その晩、夜空一面に咲く満開の花火が、ゲストの心に打ち上がった。

高齢者の旅は、寒暖差対応やトイレ誘導、食事形態など、しっかり対策しないと生命の危険を伴う。そのため、常にリスクと要望のバランスに悩まされるという。

「龍岡会では、トップに立つ理事長が"リスクを避けるよりも、ゲストに感動を与えよう"という考え。だから僕たちケアースタッフも、ゲストにとって一番よい選択をするように心がけています」。

感動するハートがあれば、いつまでも青春時代。そんな思いで、星さんはゲストのリクエストに応え続ける。

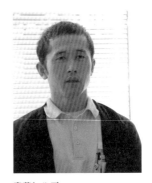

青葉ヒルズ
介護部 フロアー主任
星 英介（ほしえいすけ）
福祉大学でスポーツインストラクター学を学んだ後、療養型病院で介護職に就く。大好きだった祖母を亡くしたことをきっかけに『青葉ヒルズ』へ転職。

**Aoba Hills
Chief, Care Department
Eisuke Hoshi**

Certified care worker. After studying Sports Instruction at a Welfare University, was employed as a care nurse at a sanatorium. The loss of his beloved grandmother prompted him to move to Aoba Hills.

Endeavor in the Care Department

Lifelong Youth, Lifelong Inspiration

"I always wanted to be a professional soccer player," says Eisuke Hoshi, a member of the nursing staff at Aoba Hills. He entered the world of human care as a means of earning a living while chasing his dream and trying hard to get selected for the J-League. Now he looks back on 15 years' experience in human care. Today, as Floor Manager it is his task to coordinate his staff. One of the projects Mr. Hoshi has been involved in is a scheme to take guests outside of the facility, known as "Revisiting Favorite Places."

"A few years ago, when a guest mentioned a desire to see 'the biggest firework in Japan,' we took the plunge and organized a one-day, whirlwind trip to the Nagaoka Fireworks display in Niigata Prefecture. I'm originally from there, so I took a central role in everything, from being the driver to planning the trip. I started by making a list of the places on the way where we could eat things unique to the local area, like Shinshu *soba* noodles and *onigiri* rice balls made with *koshihikari* rice grown in Shiozawa. It's the little things that happen on the way to the destination that stick in the memory, so I thought it all through carefully, simulating every step of the journey ahead of time." That evening, the fireworks blossoming across the night sky lifted the spirits of all the guests who saw them.

"At the Tatsuoka Group, the thinking at the top, the opinion of the Chairperson, is that 'rather than avoiding risk, we should be inspiring the guests.' For that reason, the care staff do the best we can to make the best choices for the guests." A heart that can feel inspiration is forever youthful. It is this thought that keeps Mr. Hoshi responding to the requests of the guests.

介護部の取り組み
"夢見がち"なところと、"タフ"なところと

「無資格で正社員になれたのは私くらいです」と笑う、ケアースタッフの小林啓子さん。決め手は、大森理事長の「あなたは正社員で働いた方がいい」の一言だったという。「大学卒業当時は、中学・高校の国語教員になりたくて、教職浪人をしていました。その頃、仲のよい友人がヘルパーをしていたので、それで教員試験までの働き口に、と『浅草』のパート募集に申し込んだのです」。

さて、大森理事長の勧めるままに、正社員として入社を果たした小林さん。初日の研修で「故郷(ふるさと)」を合唱するゲストの姿を見て、「歴史を積み重ねてきたような重みのある歌声に胸が震えた」と感動。一方で、排泄介助の場面では、「人様のズボンを下ろすなんてこと、できません！」と抵抗し、先輩スタッフを困らせたことも。「ケアーの医学的根拠について、納得するまで看護師さんを質問攻めにしてしまったこともあります。介護の勉強をしてこなかったからこその疑問は、他のスタッフにとっては新鮮に映ったみたいです（笑）」。同期と深夜まで、介護談義に熱中することもしばしば。そんな好奇心と熱意が実を結び、『千壽』ではオープニングから介護長を務めている。

「大森理事長の"夢見がち"なところと"タフ"なところ、そしてゲストの利益にならないことはバッサリ切り捨てる潔さに、とても共感しています。介護職が子どもたちのなりたい職業No.1になることを目指して、これからも理事長と一緒に、理想の介護を究めていきたいです」。

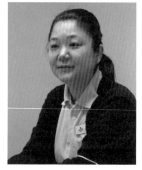

千壽介護老人保健施設
介護部 介護長
小林啓子（こばやしけいこ）
2001年に入社。『浅草』『櫻川』でケアースタッフを務めた後、現職に就く。

Endeavor in the Care Department
Both "Visionary" and "Tough"

Senju Geriatric Health Care Services Facility
Manager, Care Department
Keiko Kobayashi
Joined the Tatsuoka Group in 2001. Certified care worker, care manager. Took on her current post after working as a member of the human care staff at the Asakusa facility and the Sakuragawa facility.

"I think I'm the only permanent employee with no qualifications," laughs Keiko Kobayashi, a member of the human care staff. Her career course changed because of a comment made by Mr. Ohmori, the Chairperson: "You'd be better working as a permanent member of staff." "When I was just out of university, I wanted to become a Japanese teacher at junior high or senior high school, and instead of looking immediately for a permanent job, I decided to study for my teaching license. At that time I had a friend who was working as a helper, and thinking it would be a source of income until I could take the exam, I applied for a part-time job at the Asakusa facility."

And so on the recommendation of Mr. Ohmori, Ms. Kobayashi was able to join the Tatsuoka Group as a permanent member of staff. On the first day of training, she was moved by the sight of the guests singing "*Furusato*" (a traditional, popular children's song): "Their voices as they sang were heavy, as if they carried the weight of history in them; it made my heart pound in my chest." On the other hand, there were also times when she gave more experienced staff members a hard time; when the training involved helping a guest use the toilet she objected; "I can't pull another person's trousers down!" "There were also times when I plied the nurses with questions on the medical basis of their care, until I was satisfied with their answers. Other staff members apparently found my questions as an outsider quite refreshing," she laughs. She and the other new recruits would often stay up late at night, talking enthusiastically about human care. This curiosity and enthusiasm of hers bore fruit when Senju opened and she became its Head of Human Care.

"I totally agree with Mr. Ohmori's vision and commitment to patients. He is extremely decisive and cuts right out anything that is not to the benefit of the guests. Together with the Chairperson, I want to work towards the best possible human care, so that in the future a career in human care will be what children aspire to more than anything else."

相談部の取り組み
施設の要、ヒューマンコーディネーター

『龍岡』で相談部長を務める池田未歩さんは、今年で勤続14年目。見た目は若いが、はっきりとした口調で丁寧に話す様子に安心感を覚える。

「"悔しいかもしれないけど、今すぐ40代にはなれないし、ましてや男性にもなれないよ"。これは入社後はじめて壁にぶつかったときに、先輩から言われた言葉です。今でも、その言葉が心の支えになっています」。

施設の窓口となる相談部は、ゲストが在宅と施設のどちらに住んでも必要なサービスが整備されるように、医師や理学療法士、ケアマネージャーなど、施設内外の必要な専門家と相談をし、そのつながりをコーディネートする。

「龍岡会の相談員は、ほとんどが新卒で入職しています。そのため、ケアーの現場経験はなく、ゲストのご家族は自分の両親よりも年上の人ばかり。新人の頃は緊張のあまり、面談前はトイレにこもっていました（笑）」。

家庭の事情を明かさなければならない家族にとって、若いというだけで不信感を見せる人も少なくなかったという。カバーしきれない年齢と性別の壁。これは、龍岡会の相談員が、必ずぶつかる課題のひとつ。

「相談部長は副施設長あつかいとする」。数年前、大森理事長はあらためて全施設に通知した。家族やゲスト、さらには一緒に働くスタッフたちに、龍岡会が掲げる理念を伝える伝道者として、相談部の役割が期待された。

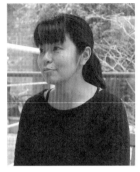

龍岡介護老人保健施設
ヒューマンコーディネーター 部長
池田未歩（いけだみほ）
2002年に入社し、2005年に部長職に就任。ケアマネージャーとしてケアプランの作成もしながら、『龍岡』の玄関口を守っている。

「私が部長になったのは 26 歳。一般の企業でも他の福祉施設でも、考えられない若さです。それでも私は、与えられた役割をまっとうしようと、若さの"メリット"に目を向けるようにしました」。

それは、パワーとフットワークの軽さに尽きる、と池田さん。パワーの源は、知識の習得とそれを体得していく現場経験の積み重ね。そして、自ら足を動かしてフロアーに上がり、ケアースタッフをはじめ他部署のスタッフたちからゲストの情報収集をするフットワーク。遠方の家族であっても、メールや電話など密なコミュニケーションを常に心がけてきた。

「珍しいスタイルですが、受付のオープンカウンターが相談員の職場ということも、情報をキャッチすることにひと役買っています。受付越しにゲストやご家族と何気なく会話する中に、ちょっとした変化が垣間見えるのです。考えてみれば、相談員は施設の窓口なので、受付に立つのは自然なことかもしれませんね」。

現在、『龍岡』の相談員は、一人約 70 人ずつ担当を持っている。決して少なくない人数を抱えていても、とくに意に介していない様子の池田さん。「協力体制ができているからなのかも。今は、ここまで任せてもらえているということにやりがいも感じています。介護は死と隣り合わせ。明るい答えが出ないこともたくさんある世界ですが、答えにたどり着くまでの過程でいかにゲストに寄り添えるか、ということを、何より大切に考えています」。

Endeavor in the Counseling Department
A Linchpin of the Facility: The Human Coordinator

This is the twelfth year Miho Ikeda, Head of the Counseling Department at the Tatsuoka facility, has been in the job. She may look young, but when she speaks, courteously and in clear tones, her words make you feel secure.

"'You may find it frustrating, but you cannot change your age, much less your gender.' This is what an older member of staff said to me the first time I hit a problem after starting work. Even today, I find inner support in those words."

The Counseling Department is the facility's liaison office, consulting specialists both within and outside the facility — doctors, physical therapists, care managers, etc. — and coordinating the connections between them to ensure that guests are provided with the services they need whether they are living at home or in the facility.

"Most the Tatsuoka Group counselors join us straight from university. This means that they have no hands-on experience of human care, and the family members of the guests are all older than their own parents. When I was a newbie, I was so nervous, I would shut myself up in a toilet cubicle before an interview," she laughs.

When it came to revealing intimate details of their family situation, not a few people, she says, were visibly distrustful of her on account of her youthfulness. Age and gender are problems that can never be fully overcome. This is one of the problems the Tatsuoka Group counselor cannot avoid coming up against.

"The Head of the Counseling Department will be looked on as the Deputy Administrator of the facility." It was some years ago that Mr. Ohmori sent out this notice to all the facilities. It was expected that the Counseling Department would take on a special mission, passing on to guests and their families, as well as to the members of staff working together, the philosophy embraced by the Tatsuoka Group.

**Tatsuoka Geriatric Health Care Services Facility Manager, Human Coordinator Department
Miho Ikeda**
Joined the Tatsuoka facility straight out of university in 2002; promoted to Head of Department in 2005. As a care manager, prepares human care plans while at the same time guarding the entrance to the Tatsuoka facility.

"I was 26 years old when I became head of the department. In any ordinary company, or even in any other welfare facility, you wouldn't imagine that happening to someone so young. Even so, I decided to focus on the 'advantages' of being young in performing the task that had been given to me."

Those advantages, according to Ms. Ikeda, boil down to energy and motivation. The source of her vigor is the knowledge she has acquired through repeated hands-on experience. And the footwork means going up in person to the floors and gathering information on the guests from not only the human care staff but also from staff in other departments. She has endeavored always to stay in close communication even with families who live far away.

"It's an unusual way of doing things, but making the open counter at Reception the place where the counselors work helps us pick up information. A casual conversation at Reception with a guest or a family member can give you a glimpse of some tiny change. When you think about it, the counselor is the contact point with the facility, so it's perhaps only natural that the counselor should be in Reception, isn't it?"

Currently, each counselor at the Tatsuoka facility is responsible for some 70 guests. This is certainly not a small number, yet it does not seem to particularly bother Ms. Ikeda. "It's probably because we have a good system of cooperation in place. Nowadays I get a sense of satisfaction from the fact that I am able to take on so much. Human care goes hand in hand with the end of life. It's a world in which there is not always a happy answer, but the most important thing for me is how closely I can relate to the guest in the process of reaching an answer."

プロジェクト部の取り組み
スタッフの満足度を高める仕掛けづくり

プロジェクト部のプロジェクトリーダー・佐藤亜希子さんは、龍岡会がスタートした1996年から勤めるベテラン社員。2004年にプロジェクト部が設立して以来、一人で業務をこなしてきた。業務内容は、スタッフの満足度を高める仕掛けづくり。法制度の改正に伴うサービス体制の変更からスタッフのストレス対処法まで、働く環境を整備する。

老人保健施設の要となる相談員からのスタート。だからこそ、大森さんとは心理的にも物理的にも距離が近く、話しやすかった。「私は新卒採用でした。当時は介護保険制度がはじまる前だったので、福祉業界は厳然たる経験者優遇の時代。相談員になるには10年の現場経験が必要だといわれていて、新卒で相談員になるのは考えられなかった。大森理事長は、その頃から新卒採用にこだわっていました」。

入社後まもなく、大森さんと2人で都庁に手続きに行った際、「お嬢さん、その若さで相談員がつとまると思っているの?」と言われたことは今でも忘れられない、と話す。そのとき大森さんは、「やれると思っているから雇っています」と、涼しい顔で答えていたという。

「理事長の理念はそれからまったく変わらない。とくに開設当時の若い頃は、頭が堅い役人の人たちに向かって、既存の枠にとらわれず、もっと介護業界全体がよくなることを取り入れていきましょうと、何度も熱く抗議していました」。

働きながら学校に行きたいと相談したときも、それが佐藤さんにとって必要なこと

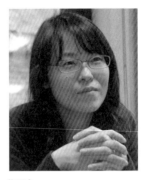

龍岡会
プロジェクト部
プロジェクトリーダー
佐藤亜希子（さとうあきこ）
大学卒業後、1996年に入社。6年後、龍岡会に在籍しながら日本女子大学大学院へ入学する。大学院での研究とケースワーカーの経験を活かし、2004年現職に就く。

であれば行きなさい、と認めた大森さん。「相談員としての経験不足を補うために、スーパーバイザーとしてベテランスタッフをつけてくれていたのですが、等身大で満足がいく対応ができず、悩んでいたときでした」。

進学先の大学院の研究テーマは「ソーシャルワーカーのストレスマネジメント」。無事に卒業できたと同時に、プロジェクト部設立の話が入り、晴れてひとりだけの部署ができた。

福祉の専門業務から管理職へ。日常業務に追われるスタッフに代わり、必要な研修や勉強会を企画したり、新しい業務体制の下地をつくる。「私の役目は基礎づくりまで。スタッフ一人ひとりに成功体験を味わってもらいたいので、個々のレベルに合わせて幅を残し、仕上げは現場に託します」。健全に働く環境であれば、みんなで助け合ってよいケアーが提供できる。そのために必要なモチベーションアップのきっかけづくりを、大切にしている。

「私が悩んだとき、理事長はいつも、佐藤さんが好きなようにやればいいんじゃない？と言ってくれます。だから、スタッフのためになることなら、自分が悩んできたことや経験を活かし、フレキシブルに取り組んでいこうと。理事長は立場上、理念を伝える役なので、現場対応に追われるスタッフと温度差が生まれることもある。私はその潤滑油になれたらいいな、と思っています」。

Endeavor in the Projects Department
Developing Ways to Raise Staff Satisfaction

Project Leader in the Projects Department, Akiko Sato is a veteran member of staff who has worked at the Tatsuoka Group ever since the start, in 1996. Since the establishment of the Projects Department in 2004, she has been a one-person section. Her job is developing ways to raise staff satisfaction. She fine-tunes the working environment; everything from making changes in the service structure following amendments to the legal system, to finding ways for staff to cope with stress.

She began work as a counselor, the linchpin in any health facility for the elderly. This is why it was easy for her to talk with Mr. Ohmori, they understand each other very well; they are psychologically and materially close. "I came here as a new graduate. At the time the long-term care insurance system had not yet been introduced, and it was a time when experience spoke volumes in the care industry. I had been told that it would take ten years of hands-on experience before I could become a counselor, and I had no thought of becoming a counselor straight out of university. But even back then, Mr. Ohmori was insisting on employing only new graduates."

She says she will never forget the time, soon after she had joined the Tatsuoka Group, when she and Mr. Ohmori went to the Tokyo Metropolitan Government building to complete some formalities and she was asked, "Miss, do you really think you can do the job of a counselor at your age? You're so young!" — to which Mr. Ohmori had replied with studied indifference, "I hired her because I knew she could do the job."

"The Chairperson's philosophy has not changed at all since then. In particular at the time the facility opened, when we were still young, he had numerous heated arguments with stubborn civil servants, saying that they should be doing more to improve the human care industry as a whole, instead of being shackled by the existing rigid framework."

The Tatsuoka Group
Projects Department
Project Leader
Akiko Sato
Joined the Tatsuoka Group as a care manager in 1996, after graduating from university. Six years later, entered the Graduate School of the Japan Women's University and undertook her studies while remaining an employee of the Tatsuoka Group. In 2004 took up her present position, where she puts her master's degree in Social Work and her experience as a welfare officer to good use.

When Ms. Sato discussed with him the possibility of her going back to school while working, Mr. Ohmori gave his approval, telling her that if she thought it necessary, she should go to school. "In order to cover my lack of experience as a counselor, he put a veteran member of staff in place as my supervisor, but at the time I was worried that I wasn't able to manage things candidly and satisfactorily." Her postgraduate research theme was "Stress Management for Social Workers." Just at the time that she completed her studies without incident, talk of establishing a Projects Department came up, and she became the only member of her very own Department.

From specialist welfare services to management. On behalf of the staff members who are caught up in their everyday duties, she plans the training and seminars they need and lays the groundwork for new working structures. "My work stops at the building of the foundation. We want each member of staff to enjoy the taste of success, so I leave some latitude commensurate with the level of the individual, and leave it up to the people doing the work to finish things off."

If the working environment is sound, everyone can work together to provide better human care. She concentrates on creating opportunities to raise everyone's motivation.

"Whenever I'm worried, the Chairperson always says, 'You should do as you think best.' So if it's something that will benefit the staff, I decide to tackle things flexibly, turning what I was worried about to advantage and capitalizing on my experience. In his position, the role of the Chairperson is to get his principles across, and sometimes the staff members who are working in the front line might have different concerns. If I can act as a lubricant between the two, then I've done my job."

栄養部の取り組み
思い出の料理をもう一度

"あなたにとって、懐かしい料理は何ですか?"。栄養部の今井敦子さんは、『青葉ヒルズ』に入居したゲストに問いかける。「ゲストとお話していると、必ずといっていいほど、思い出話の中に食べ物が登場します。その味はその人にとって、いつまでも色褪せない。大人になって口にしたときに、懐かしくて心が温かくなるような思い出の味の再現が、私の使命です」。

今井さんの担当は、龍岡会独自の取り組み「ハーティーミール®＝心のこもった食事」。毎日の献立をつくるのではなく、看取りに近いゲストが、最期にもう一度食べたい料理を再現する。その場合、ゲストの多くは通常の食事形態がむずかしい身体状況のため、料理を一度ミキサーで粉砕してから、味や形を組み立てていくことも。前職が介護食の開発に携わっていた今井さんだからこそ、実現可能な技といえる。

あるとき、お家が和菓子店を営んでいた93歳の女性ゲストが、「子どもの頃に食べていたお饅頭をもう一度食べたい」とつぶやいた。確認すると、ゲストの和菓子店は、とうに店を閉めているという。条件は、皮が薄くて口当たりがよい、漉し餡入り。今井さんは、嚥下障害があるそのゲストでも食べることができるお饅頭を、さっそくリサーチ。まずは看護師に試食してもらう。「うん、これなら心配ない。食べても大丈夫よ」。医療の専門家にチェックを受けて、身体的な問題はクリアできた。あとは口に入れた瞬間に、懐かしい思い出とリンクするか、それが肝心だ。ドキドキしながら、ゲストにお饅頭を差し出す。

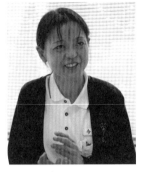

青葉ヒルズ
管理栄養士
今井敦子（いまいあつこ）
病院栄養士を6年半務めた後、企業で介護食品の営業・開発に携わる。2009年に入社。モットーは、"常識にとらわれない美味しい介護食"の提供。

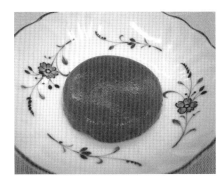

煎餅
煎餅のソフト食。味が濃くて香ばしいたまり醤油の煎餅をミルサーにかけ、噛み砕いて飲み込むときの食感を再現した

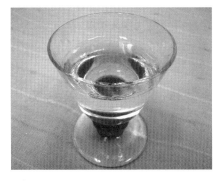

日本酒ゼリー
日本酒が大好きなゲストのために。煮てアルコールを抜き、少し甘さを加えて固める。食感はスルッとした喉越し、切子のお猪口で雰囲気を演出

「美味しい！うちのお饅頭の味がする！」。ひとくち食べて、ゲストの顔がほころんだ。「ゲストの笑顔と"ありがとう"の言葉をいただくと、栄養士冥利に尽きます。実はそのゲストは、お饅頭を食べた1週間後にお亡くなりに……。ご家族にそのお話をご報告したら、母がそんな昔のことを覚えていたなんて、とびっくりされていました」。

他にも、水を加えない関西風のすきやきや、香ばしい香りがするソフト食のお煎餅、江戸っ子向けのあまじょっぱいみたらし団子など、今井さん作の再現料理は数知れず。一度目で「違う」と言われ、二度三度と挑戦したこともある。「当時と同じお煎餅の堅さや、すき焼きの味付けの濃さでは、思い出とリンクしないのです。今のゲストの状態で同じように美味しく食べられるものをつくることが、何よりむずかしい」と話す。

「今だ！と思ったときにすぐに実行しないと、ゲストの病状が悪化して何も食べられない状態になってしまうことも。でも、重度の認知症で色々なことがわからなくなっていても、口からの刺激は残っている場合もあるんです」。

ゲストが最期に呼び起こしたい風景が、思い出の味から広がっていく―。それは、今井さん流の回想療法といえる。

Endeavor in the Nutrition Department
A Taste of Nostalgia

"What are the foods that you have good memories of?" Atsuko Imai of the Nutrition Department asks new guests to Aoba Hills. "When we're talking to a guest, almost without fail food will make an appearance in their reminiscences. For that person, the memory of that taste is something that will never fade away. My job is to recreate those nostalgic, heart-warming flavors that bring back memories with each mouthful."

Ms. Imai is in charge of "Hearty Meals®," an initiative unique to the Tatsuoka Group. This is not the creation of the daily menu, but the recreation, for guests near the end of their time, of the food they want to eat one more time in their final days. In such situations, many guests are not able to enjoy their food in the normal way; sometimes the food has to be pureed in a blender and arranged to recreate the taste and shape. Thanks to her previous experience in developing human care meals, Ms. Imai is perhaps just the person to make this possible.

At one time, a 93-year-old lady guest whose family had once run a Japanese confectionery store mentioned that she would like once more to eat the sweet steamed bean-jam bun she had eaten as a child. A quick check revealed that the family store had closed down long ago. The bun in question had a thin outer covering encasing smooth bean jam that was pleasant to the palate. Ms. Imai immediately set out researching bean-jam buns to find one that the guest, who had trouble swallowing, could enjoy. First of all, she got the nurse to try it. "Mmm, this is OK. She will have no trouble eating this." Next, she got a medical expert to check it and got the all-clear; the bun would pose no physical problems for the guest. All that remained was the question of whether when the guest tasted the bun, it would bring back the taste she remembered. Nervously, she offered the bun to the guest.

Aoba Hills
Registered Dietitian
Atsuko Imai
After working for six and a half years as a hospital dietitian, was engaged in the commercial marketing/development of human care foods. Joined the Tatsuoka Group in 2009. Her motto is "Delicious human care food not fettered by convention."

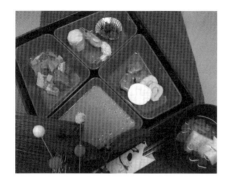

Special dishes for New Year's
We've recreated New Year's traditional dishes using soft food. Doing our best to recreate the original look and delicious taste, we use a mixer and gelling agents to get the food as close as possible to the original.

At the first taste, the guest's face lit up. "This is so good! It tastes just like the buns we used to have at our store!"

"Seeing a smile on the guest's face and hearing the words 'Thank you' — this is what makes me glad I became a nutritionist. In fact, the guest mentioned earlier passed away a week after eating the bean-jam bun. When I related the story to the family, they were surprised that their mother had remembered things from so long ago."

In addition to the sweet bean-jam bun, there are numerous foods Ms. Imai has recreated: Kansai-style *sukiyaki*, to which water is not added; fragrant rice crackers that melt in the mouth; the salty-sweet *mitarashi-dango* skewered rice dumplings favored by long-established Tokyoites. Sometimes her first attempts have been met with "No, that's not it," and she went back to try a second or third time. "Rice crackers as hard as the ones they ate in the past, or *sukiyaki* with the same depth of seasoning, doesn't match their memories. There is nothing as difficult as making something that the guests can enjoy now in their present state, just as much as they used to in the past," she says.

"If you don't act when the time is right, sometimes the guest's condition can deteriorate to the point where they cannot eat anything. That said, it often happens that even when a person has severe dementia and no longer understands all kinds of things, that person is still able to appreciate taste."

Expanding a guest's vista in the final days via the unforgettable tastes of the past, this is reminiscence therapy, Imai-style.

アート部の取り組み
人生にアートは欠かせない

「作品を見て、はじめて義母の気持ちが見えた気がします」。認知症のゲストがプログラムで描いた絵を見て、過去のわだかまりが消えたと話す娘さん。「作品に表現されたリズムや色彩から、ゲストを多角的に見ることができるのは、アートの面白いところです」。アート部長の石川温子さんが穏やかに答えた。

アート部の活動は、施設の中で特別な存在。"専門家による本格的なセラピー"は、龍岡会のサービス精神「ハーティケアー＝心が癒される、誠心誠意のケアー」を支えている。

「"美術の視点からケアーをしてくれる人を募集します"。大学に張り出された求人広告を見つけて、飛びつきました。元々介護の道に進もうと考えていたのですが、美術大学で学んだ知識も活かせるなんて、めったにないチャンスですから」。

たしかに、介護施設で本格的なセラピーを行うときは、外部からセラピストを呼ぶことが多く、常勤で採用するケースはあまり例がない。しかも、お金を集めて手厚いサービスが提供できるような民間企業ではなく、龍岡会は非営利団体だ。

「入居された人がまず求めるものは、衣食住のケアー。私たちは、身体面の活性化を図るリハビリとも少し異なり、気持ちの活性化が中心の活動です。きちんと目標を立てて段階的にプログラムを実施していくことで、ゲストの集中力を高めたり、自信回復を図ります。生活に根ざしたアートだからこそ、心が豊かになり、暮らしに潤いが生まれる。龍岡会独自のこの取り組みを、私たちスタッフも誇りに感じています」。

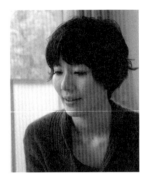

龍岡会
アート部 部長
石川温子（いしかわあつこ）
2008年に多摩美術大学油絵科卒業後、おばあちゃん・おじいちゃんっ子だったこともあり、現職に就く。「アートで社会とのつながりを、もっと広げていきたい」。

アート部の活動は、美術と音楽の2つの領域に分かれている。それぞれ専属スタッフが一日1〜1.5時間枠のプログラムを3つ程度実施し、ゲストの変化や上達を記録に残す。プログラムは、個別対応から10人以上の集団レクリエーションまで様々。とくに音楽では、個別療法に力を入れている。

「暮らしの視点からセラピーを実施できるのは、龍岡会ならでは。ご家族やケアーマネージャー、フロアーのケアースタッフと目標を共有して、回復過程を観察していきます。例えば、失語症で言葉を発することがむずかしいけれど歌うことはできる、というゲストには、メロディーにあわせて"おはよう"の歌唱練習からスタート。その内容を、ゲストのそばにいるケアースタッフと共有することで、普段の挨拶へとスムーズにつなげていくことができるのです」。

これからの課題は、科学的な裏付けが少ないアートの世界で、セラピー効果をevidence（証明）していくこと。「美術のアクティビティは認知症ケア学会で、音楽セラピーは音楽療法学会でそれぞれ発表を行っていて、音楽の研究発表は、3年に1度開催される世界大会で発表しました。龍岡会のポリシーのひとつに「"Care Science® = 介護を科学すること"」という言葉があります。暮らしに寄り添うアートの大切さを証明するため、これからも外部に向けて発信していきたいですね」。

Endeavor in the Art Department
Art is an Indispensable Part of Life

"When I saw what my mother-in-law had drawn, I felt that for the first time I could understand how she felt." Seeing the picture a guest with dementia had drawn as part of the program, her daughter-in-law spoke of how all the ill feeling from the past disappeared. Atsuko Ishikawa, Head of the Art Department, responded gently, "The interesting thing about art is that the rhythm and coloring in a picture allows us to see the guest from a number of different angles."

The activities of the Art Department occupy a special position within the facility. "Authentic therapy by specialists" supports the Tatsuoka Group spirit of good service illustrated in the motto "Heartfelt care = Whole-hearted, devoted, compassionate human care."

"'Vacancy for person able to provide human care from the perspective of art.' When I came across this notice on the university situations-vacant bulletin board, I jumped at the chance. I'd been considering making my career in human care all along, but this was a rare opportunity to make the most of what I had studied at art university, which I hadn't expected." It is true that when a human care facility provides authentic therapy classes, in most cases the therapist is brought in from outside; there are not many instances of a therapist being employed full-time. Add to that the fact that the Tatsuoka Group is not a private-sector business enterprise that is able to take in money in order to be able to provide convivial, generous services, but a non-profit organization.

"What the people who come to live at the facility want first of all is to have the basic needs of food, clothing and shelter met. What we do is a little bit different from rehabilitation, which aims to revitalize a person physically; our activities center instead on revitalizing a person's state of mind. By setting precise goals and implementing the program step by step, we work to improve the guests' powers of concentration and to restore their self-confidence. It is because it is

The Tatsuoka Group
Head of Department, Art Department
Atsuko Ishikawa
After graduating in Oil Painting from Tama Art University in 2008, took up employment in her present post, influenced in part by her closeness to her own grandparents. "I want to expand social interaction through art."

art that is rooted in life that it opens up the mind and adds interest to daily life. This initiative is unique to the Tatsuoka Group, and is something we members of staff all feel proud of."

The activities of the Art Department are divided into two segments: fine art, and music. In both art and music, a specialist member of staff runs three programs or so a day, in sessions lasting one to one and a half hours each, and records any changes or improvements noticed in each guest. The programs are varied, from one-on-one sessions to group recreation sessions for ten or more participants. In music in particular, the emphasis is on personalized therapy.

"Carrying out therapy from the perspective of daily life is something at which the Tatsuoka Group excels. Family members as well as the care manager and human care staff working on the floor all share the same goal, and observe the process of recovery closely. For example, for a guest with aphasia who finds speaking difficult but is able to sing, we start by practicing singing the words 'Good morning' to a melody. The human care staff member who is sitting with the guest can share this and use it to lead smoothly into ordinary everyday greetings."

A challenge that still remains is proving the effectiveness of therapy in the world of art, for which there is as yet little scientific support. "We have given presentations on art activities at the Japanese Society for Dementia Care, and on music therapy at the Japanese Music Therapy Association, and we have given a music presentation at the World Congress held once every three years. The Tatsuoka Group policy includes the words, 'Care Science® = the Science of Long-Term Care.' I want to continue telling the outside world about our activities, in order to demonstrate the importance of art as an integral part of daily life."

アート部の取り組み
大手ホテルでの展覧会

過去2回ほど大手ホテルで開催した展覧会は、ゲストにとってもスタッフにとっても、思い出に残る一大イベントだった。

「1998年にホテルオークラで開催された展覧会は、お忍びで皇后陛下美智子様が来られました。当時では珍しい取り組みだったので、新聞に取り上げられたのです。会場は1000人以上の来館者で大賑わい。他の介護施設の見本になれたら、という思いもありました。日の目を見ない介護業界の活性化を、強く願っていた時代のことです」（大森さん）。

2011年に帝国ホテルで開催した2度目の展覧会では、アート部のスタッフが大活躍。龍岡会全施設のゲストの作品を集めた結果、個性豊かな芸術品が会場を飾った。

「このとき大切にしていたのは、普段なかなか面会に来られないご家族も巻き込んで、みんなで達成感を味わうこと」。そう懐かしそうに話す、アート部の石川さん。当日は、会場を訪れる人が目を輝かせて作品を眺めている姿に大満足。「半年かけて、準備した甲斐がありました（笑）」。

アートのよいところは、"形に残せること"と石川さん。「忘れがちだけど、ゲストは年齢的に死に近いところにいる。いつ最期の作品になってしまうかわからないからこそ、今この瞬間にどれだけ感動できるか、それを専門家として導いていきたい」。

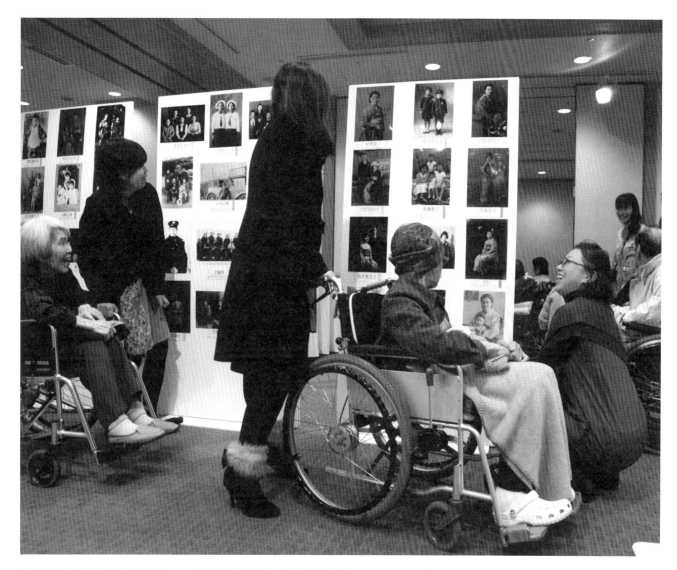

ゲストの生きた記録を一覧にまとめた、100年にわたる写真年表。「施設で生活を共にしているゲストが、中学時代は同じ土地で暮らし、その後、ひとりは東京を離れ、ひとりはずっとそこに残り……。それぞれの人生がクロスして、再び龍岡会で縁を結ぶ。人のつながりが目で追えるので面白かったです」（石川さん）

Endeavor in the Art Department
Exhibitions at Leading Hotels

Exhibitions at leading hotels have been held twice in the past, and for both guests and staff, these exhibitions have been memorable events.
"The exhibition held at the Hotel Okura in 1998 was attended incognito by Her Imperial Highness the Empress Michiko. It was a rare event at the time, and it was reported in the newspapers. The exhibition had a very good turnout, with over a thousand visitors. We hoped that it would set an example for other human care facilities. It was a time when the world of human care was largely unknown, and we strongly desired to give it stimulation." (Mr. Ohmori)
At the second exhibition, held in 2011 at the Imperial Hotel, the staff of the Art Department worked very hard. Thanks to their efforts in collecting works from guests at all of the Tatsuoka Group facilities, the venue was adorned with very distinctive works of art.
"What we focused on then was involving family members who normally have difficulty coming to see the guests, so that everyone could share in the feeling of a job well done," says Ms. Ishikawa, a nostalgic tone in her voice. She says she felt great satisfaction on the day of the exhibition, seeing the visitors' eyes shining as they viewed the exhibits. "We'd spent half a year getting things ready, and seeing that made it all worthwhile," she laughs.
The good thing about art, says Ms. Ishikawa, is that it "leaves behind something concrete." "It's something we tend to forget," she says, "but in terms of age, the guests are close to the end of their lives. It is exactly because we do not know which work will turn out to be their last that as a professional therapist I want to guide them towards feeling as much emotion as possible in what they are doing now."

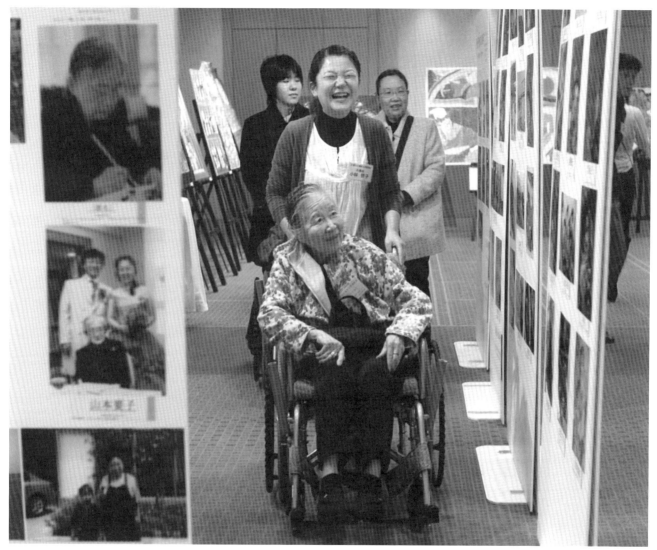

A timeline in photos, bringing together a record of guests' lives over a period of a hundred years. "Guests now living together in the facility lived in the same area when they were young; after leaving school, one moved away from Tokyo, while the other remained here the whole time... Their lives intersected, and they renewed their friendship at the Tatsuoka Group. It was interesting having a visible trace of the connections between people." (Ms. Ishikawa)

医療への取り組み
暮らしを支える町の診療所

「老人保健施設は、"治療の場"ではなく"暮らしの場"に近い。だから、暮らしの主役はゲストで、暮らしを支えるケアーの中心は、介護士や看護師のスタッフです」。そう話すのは、『龍岡』の施設長であり、『大森医院』の院長でもある石川みずえ医師。

「家庭医(ホームドクター)」と「施設長」の2つの顔を持つ石川医師の一日は慌しい。大森医院で外来診療を行い、近隣の家へ訪問診療に向かう。それに加えて、『龍岡』の回診もある。この地域では、『大森医院』で診断を受けて『龍岡』に入所する人もいれば、『龍岡』でリハビリを終えて自宅に戻り、『大森医院』に通う人もいる。昭和初期の診療所の姿を今も守っている『大森医院』の存在が、「地域包括ケア」の要となっているのだ。

体ひとつでは足りないようなスケジュールをこなす石川医師。だが、「『龍岡』のことは、現場のスタッフがしっかりゲストを見ているから安心している」という。「相談業務、リハビリ、ケアーなど、ここのスタッフは専門家の集団です。だから、施設長としての私の仕事は、"最終的に責任を持つこと"。ゲストにとって前向きなことであれば、ダメなことは何ひとつとしてないのが医療現場とは違うところ。だから、スタッフは各自で判断をして、自由に動いて欲しいと思っています。スタッフがやりがいを持ち、笑顔で働く職場であれば、ゲストも笑顔になる。『龍岡』での医師としての役割は、治療ではなく、必要なときに道しるべになることなのです」。

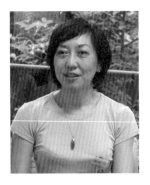

大森医院 院長
龍岡介護老人保健施設 施設長
石川みずえ

日本医科大学医学部卒業。医学博士。産婦人科医を経て、2000年『浅草』の施設長に就く。大森理事長の父が亡くなった後、『龍岡』の施設長と大森医院を引き継ぐ。

Endeavor in Medical Care

The Town Clinic at the Center of Local Life

Director, Ohmori Clinic
Director, Tatsuoka Geriatric Health Care Services Facility
Mizue Ishikawa (M.D., Ph.D.)

Graduated from Nippon Medical School. Doctor of Medicine. After working in obstetrics and gynecology, in 2000 took up the post of Facility Director at the Asakusa facility. After the passing of Mr. Ohmori's father, became Facility Director at the Tatsuoka facility and Director of the Ohmori Clinic.

"A geriatric health care services facility is not so much a place of treatment as a part of daily life. As such, it is the guests who play the leading role in the daily life of the facility, and the staff — the care workers and nurses — who are at the center of the human care that supports that daily life." These are the words of Dr. Mizue Ishikawa, Facility Director at the Tatsuoka facility and Director of the Ohmori Clinic. With two hats to wear — as a family physician and as a facility director — Dr. Ishikawa's days are busy. After holding her outpatients medical examinations at the Ohmori Clinic, she goes out on house calls in the local area. In addition to this, she has her rounds at the Tatsuoka facility to attend to. In this area, there are people who move into the Tatsuoka facility after being diagnosed at the Ohmori Clinic as well as people who, after completing rehabilitation at the Tatsuoka facility, return to their own homes and receive outpatient care at the Ohmori Clinic. Founded in the early Showa Era (late 1920s), the Ohmori Clinic has played an essential role in comprehensive nursing care in the community.

Dr. Ishikawa gets through a schedule so full it's hard to imagine any one person could manage. But, she says, "The staff at the Tatsuoka facility keep a very close and careful eye on the guests, and I have every confidence in them. The staff, whether they be engaged in consultation, rehabilitation, human care or whatever, are all experts in their field. So my job as Facility Director is to just to be the person who is ultimately responsible. Where we differ from a medical facility is that nothing is ever ruled out, so long as it's positive for the guest. This is why my thinking is that I want the staff to make their own decisions and to be free to act as they see fit. When a staff member feels the job they are doing is worthwhile, and they can work with a smile on their face, that puts a smile on the guest's face, too. My role as a doctor at the Tatsuoka Group facilities is primarily to act as a guide when necessary, not to provide medical treatment."

スタッフの海外研修
五感で学ぶ

海外留学を経験した大森さんによる、スペシャル研修。それは、スタッフたちと一緒に、外国の介護施設を見学すること。大森さんは、海外文化にふれることが情操教育やスタッフの見聞を広め、よいケアーにつながると考えている。

「毎年8名ほどスタッフを連れて行きます。見学先のアポ取りから現地の運転手、通訳まで、すべて私がアテンド。ノルウェー、スウェーデン、デンマーク、イギリス、ドイツ、と、9日で5カ国巡ったこともありますよ」。

日中は見学、夜はみんなでミーティングという、目が回るようなハードスケジュール。手づくり感満載の研修は、いつも多くの思い出を胸に刻んだという。

「最初に実施したのは1998年。ワーキングエキスチェンジとして、スタッフをひとり現地に送り込み、その国からひとりスタッフを迎え入れる。海外で働く経験をしてもらいました。でも、言葉の壁がネックになってしまい、今は私が引率して、みんなで行くようになりました」。

毎年ホームステイでお世話になっているご夫婦のご主人が亡くなったときは、「ご主人のお墓参りと、ひとりになってしまった奥様と思い出話を語ろう」と、縁のあるスタッフたちを誘い、訪ねたこともある。

「とても勉強になりましたが体力的にはへとへと……。一方、理事長はずっと元気で、目をキラキラさせてアテンドしてくれました（笑）」とは、研修から帰国したスタッフ談。「アカデミックなことに力をいれたい」と語る、教育熱心な大森さんのガイド姿が目に浮かぶ。

2012年、デンマークにて。JJW建築事務所設計の有料老人ホームを視察

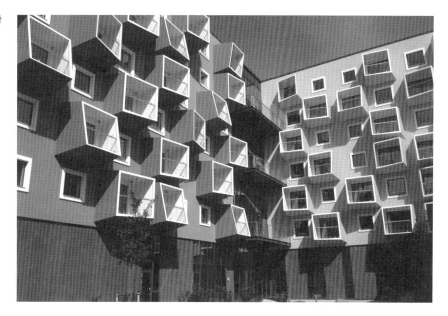

日照時間が少ない北欧では、日光浴しながらのティータイムが毎日の楽しみだそう

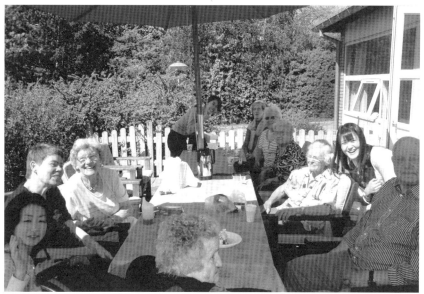

Overseas Staff Training
Learning Through the Five Senses

This is special training undertaken by Mr. Ohmori, who has experience of studying abroad. This special training involves visits by the staff and Mr. Ohmori to human care facilities outside Japan. It is Mr. Ohmori's belief that coming into contact with different cultures leads to better human care through the cultivation of esthetic sensibilities and the enrichment of the staff's stock of knowledge.
"Every year I take around eight members of staff with me. I take care of everything from making appointments at the places we are going to visit, to driving us around and interpreting. On one trip we took in five countries — Norway, Sweden, Denmark, the UK and Germany — in nine days."
The schedule is dizzying; touring facilities during the daytime, and meetings attended by everyone in the evenings. The study tour has a home-made feel to it, and the journey always yields a harvest of stirring memories in our hearts.
"The first overseas training took place in 1998. It was a working exchange; we sent one member of our staff abroad, and in exchange took in one staff member from that country. The idea was to have the staff experience working abroad. However, the language barrier proved to be a problem. These days I take a whole group overseas."
When the husband of a couple in Denmark who had welcomed the Tatsuoka Group staff into their home every year passed away, Mr. Ohmori invited members of staff who knew the couple to go with him to visit the husband's grave, and talk over old times with his widow.
Staff who have been on one of the overseas trips say laughingly, "It was very informative, but physically exhausting…but the Chairperson was always full of energy, and looked after us with a twinkle in his eye." We can just picture Mr. Ohmori, with his enthusiasm for education, saying "I want us to focus on academic matters more than care techniques," as he acts as tour guide.

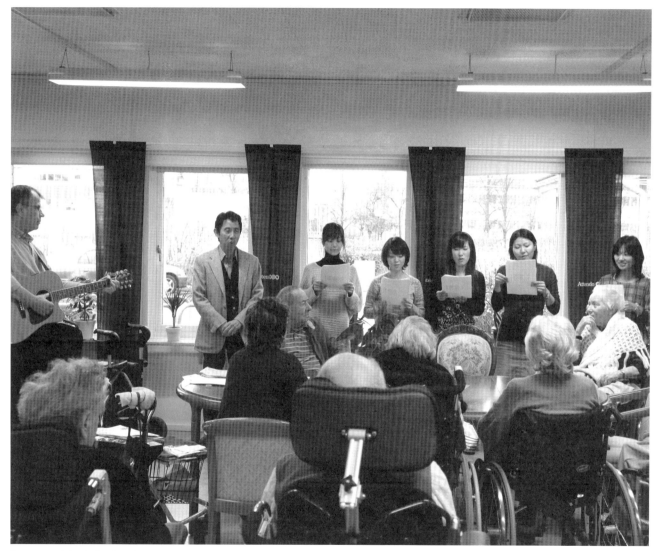

Overseas training in Northern Europe
Singing "Itomaki no uta," which was originally a Danish folk song, to cheer everyone up

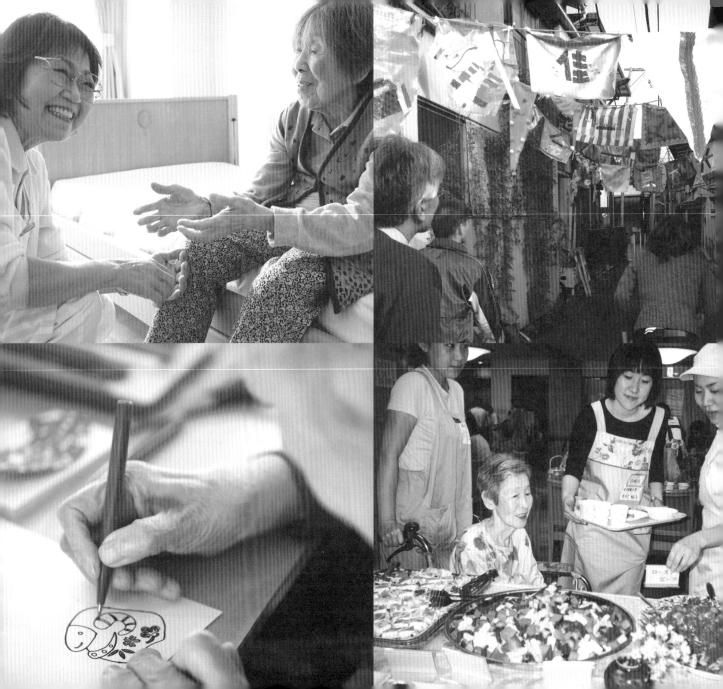

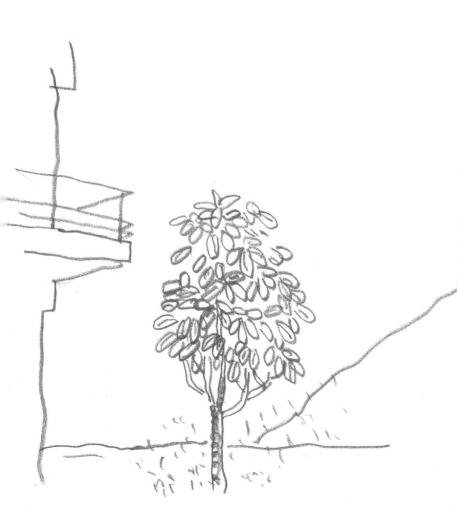

施設紹介
龍岡介護老人保健施設
浅草介護老人保健施設
櫻川介護老人保健施設
神石介護老人保健施設
千壽介護老人保健施設
千壽グループホーム
ワセダグループホーム
青葉ヒルズ(特別養護老人ホーム)

Facilities
Tatsuoka Geriatric Health Care Services Facility
Asakusa Geriatric Health Care Services Facility
Sakuragawa Geriatric Health Care Services Facility
Kamiishi Geriatric Health Care Services Facility
Senju Geriatric Health Care Services Facility
Senju Group Home
Waseda Group Home
Aoba Hills (Special Nursing Home)

龍岡介護老人保健施設
Tatsuoka Geriatric Health Care Services

山手線環内にはじめて設立された都市型の介護老人保健施設。龍岡会創立の地である文京区湯島にあり、緑あふれる東京大学や上野公園にほど近く、静かな環境。生活そのものがリハビリテーションとなるよう、施設のつくりやプログラムなどに配慮がなされている。

This was the first urban geriatric health care services facility for the elderly within the Yamanote Line area in Tokyo. It is located in the Yushima section of Bunkyo ward where the Tatsuoka Group was founded, in a quiet, wooded neighborhood close to Tokyo University and Ueno Park. The facility's structure and programs are designed so that daily life itself becomes a rehabilitating experience.

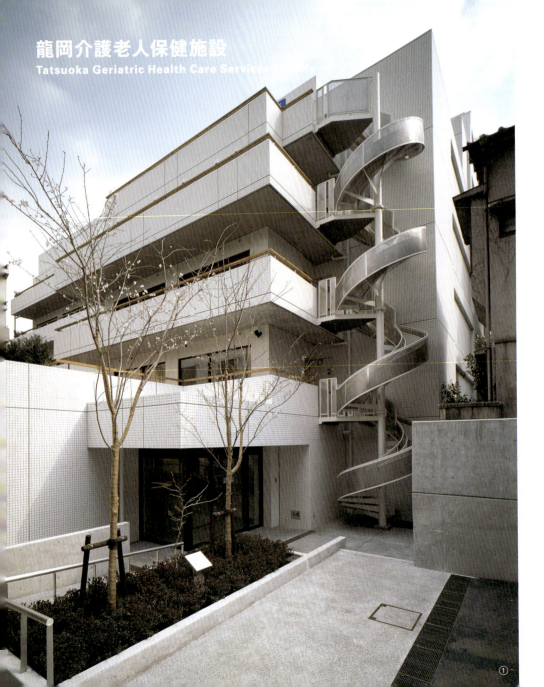
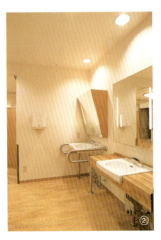

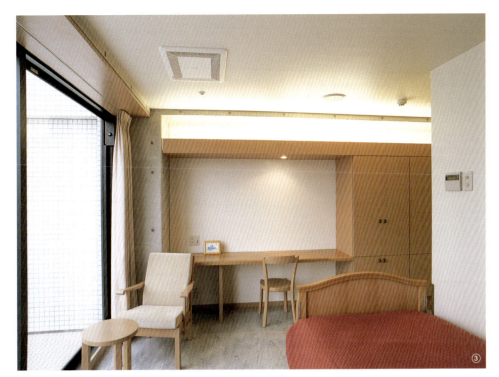
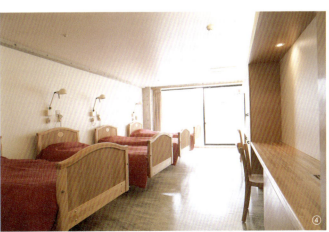
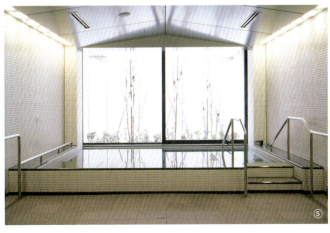

龍岡介護老人保健施設
入所（短期含む）：100名
通所リハビリ：50名
施設：4人室、2人室、個室
〒113-0034 東京都文京区湯島 4-9-8
TEL. 03-3811-0088

Tatsuoka Geriatric Health Care Services Facility
Long-stay & short-stay: 100 guests
Day-care(rehabilitation): 50 guests
Type of rooms: Four-person, double, and private
4-9-8 Yushima, Bunkyo-ku, Tokyo 113-0034
Tel.: 03-3811-0088

① 外観 Exterior view
② 洗面室 Washroom
③ 個室 Private room
④ 4人室 Four-person room
⑤ 浴室 Bathroom

施設紹介 Facilities

浅草介護老人保健施設
Asakusa Geriatric Health Care Services Facility

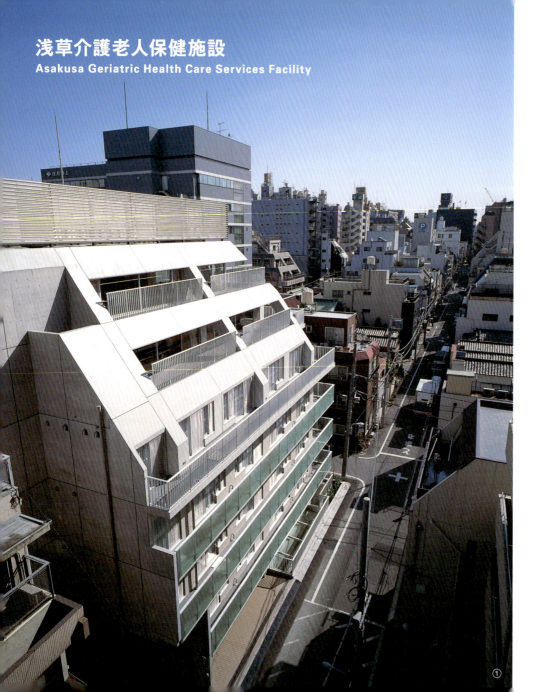

浅草寺に近く、アクセスに便利な街中にある施設。大きなテラスや屋上からは、浅草三社祭や隅田川の花火大会などを楽しめる。木のぬくもりを活かした明るい印象の内装で、ゲストやリハビリテーション利用者は、日常の暮らしに近い感覚で過ごすことができる。

The Asakusa facility is located in an easy-to-access downtown area near the Senso-ji Temple. From the spacious terrace and rooftop, guests can enjoy the Asakusa Sanja Matsuri, the Sumida River Fireworks Festival, and many other events. With its warm, cheery wooden interior, the facility allows guests and outpatients to have normal everyday lifestyles.

① 外観 Exterior view
② 4人室 Four-person room
③ ロビー Lobby
④ リハビリ室 Rehabilitation Room
⑤ 浴室 Bathroom

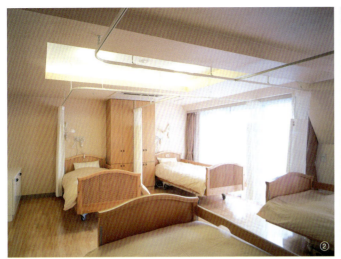
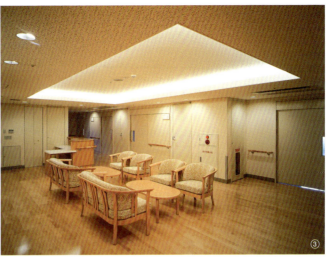
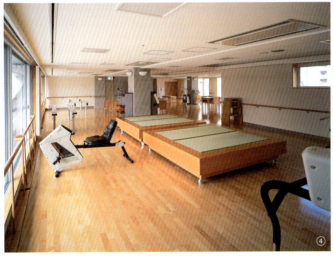
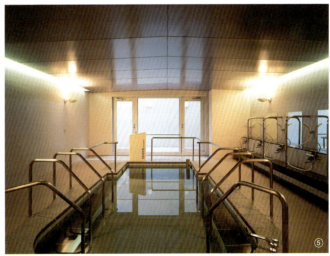

浅草介護老人保健施設
入所（短期含む）：100名
通所リハビリ：40名
施設：4人室、3人室
〒111-0042 東京都台東区寿 4-8-2
TEL. 03-5806-0088

Asakusa Geriatric Health Care Services Facility
Long-stay & short-stay: 100 guests
Day-care(rehabilitation): 40 guests
Type of rooms: Four-person and three-person
4-8-2 Kotobuki, Taito-ku, Tokyo 111-0042
Tel.: 03-5806-0088

櫻川介護老人保健施設
Sakuragawa Geriatric Health Care Services Facility

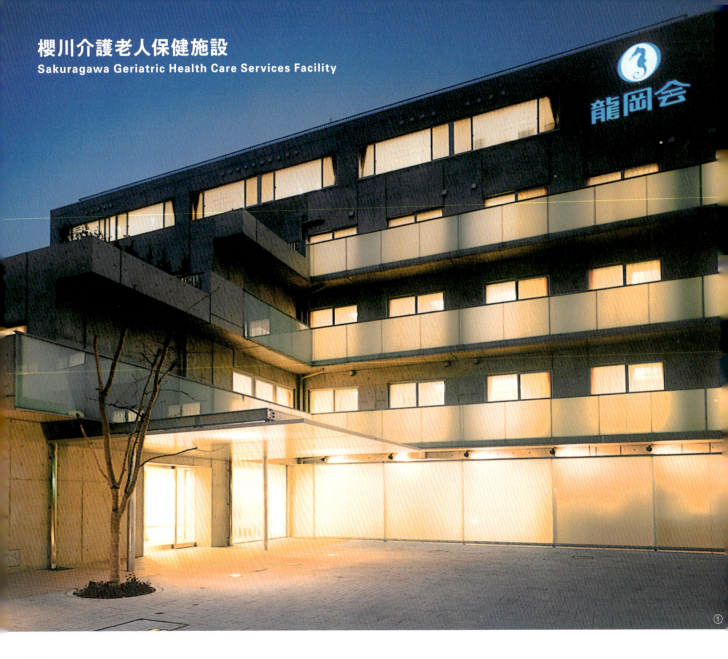

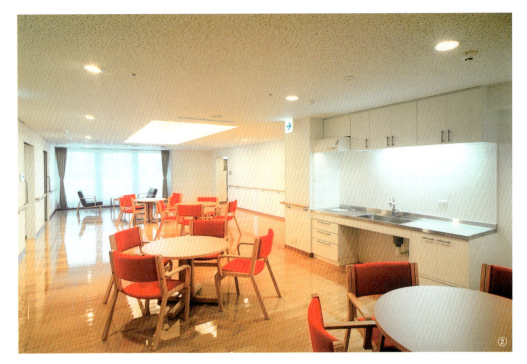

隅田川を臨む場所に位置し、周囲を緑に囲まれた施設。大きな窓からは明るい光が差し込み、お花見や花火大会を楽しむなど、季節を感じながら過すことができる。それぞれにキッチンを備えたユニット式の設えで、ゲストの自主性と快適性を尊重する家庭的なケアーをおこなっている。

Surrounded by trees and overlooking the Sumida River, the Sakuragawa facility has large windows that let in lots of sunlight and that provide excellent views of cherry blossoms, fireworks displays, and more. Living here, guests spend their time in touch with the seasons. Individual units are furnished with their own kitchens and a home-like style of care is provided out of respect for the independence and comfort of guests.

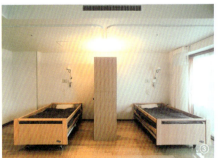
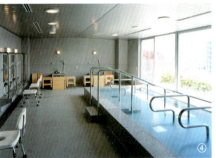
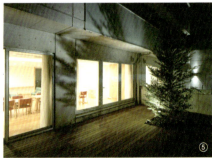

櫻川介護老人保健施設
入所（短期含む）：152 名
通所リハビリ：30 名
施設：4人室
〒131-0034 東京都墨田区堤通 1-9-8
TEL. 03-5630-0088

Sakuragawa Geriatric Health Care Services Facility
Long-stay & short-stay: 152 guests
Day-care (rehabilitation): 30 guests
Type of rooms: Four-person
1-9-8 Tsutsumidori, Sumida-ku, Tokyo 131-0034
Tel.: 03-5630-0088

① エントランス夜景 Entrance night view
② ユニットルーム Unit rooms
③ 4人室 Four-person room
④ 浴室 Bathroom
⑤ テラス夜景 Terrace at night

施設紹介 Facilities 127

神石介護老人保健施設
Kamiishi Geriatric Health Care Services Facility

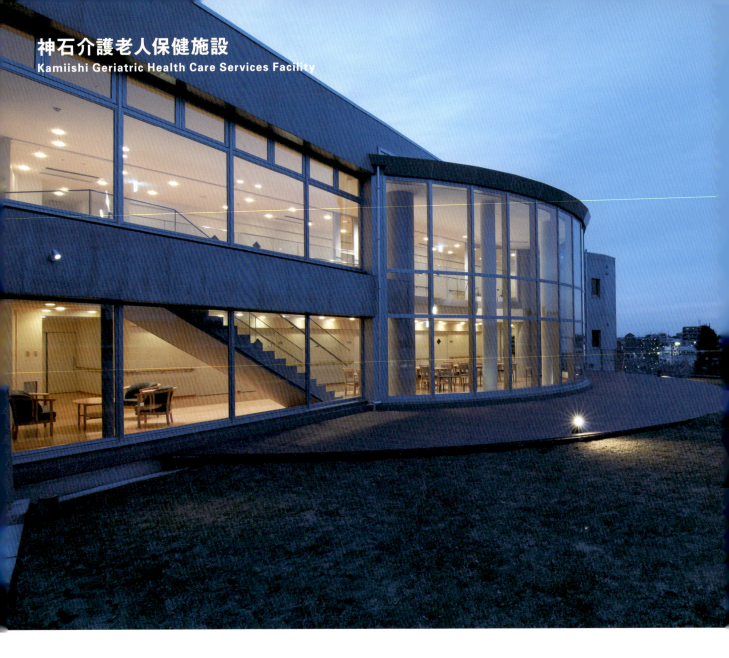

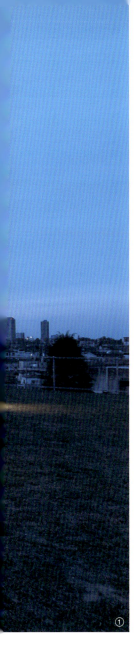
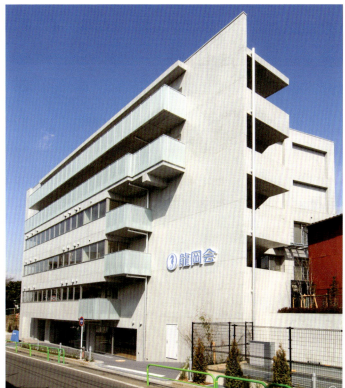
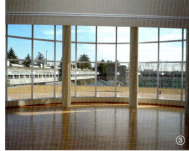
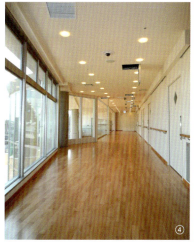

武蔵野の面影を深く残す石神井に位置し、石神井公園の豊かな緑を感じながらゆったりと過すことができる。都心に隣接したアクセスのよさと、季節のうつろいを感じられる自然とが共存した恵まれた環境で、それぞれのゲストのペースに寄り添うケアーをおこなっている。

Located in Shakujii, which preserves the spirit of Musashino, the Kamiishi facility allows guests to relax and enjoy the lush greenery of Shakujii Park. The facility has easy access to the nearby downtown area and a comfortable environment that allows guests to be in sync with nature and the seasons. Nursing care that perfectly matches the pace of each guest is provided.

神石介護老人保健施設
入所（短期含む）：123 名
通所リハビリ：36 名
施設：4 人室、個室
〒177-0044 東京都練馬区上石神井 3-33-6
TEL. 03-3594-0088

Kamiishi Geriatric Health Care Services Facility
Long-stay & short-stay: 123 guests
Day-care (rehabilitation): 36 guests
Type of rooms: Four-person and private
3-33-6 Kamishakujii, Nerima-ku, Tokyo 177-0044
Tel.: 03-3594-0088

① 外観夜景 Exterior night view　② 外観 Exterior view　③ レクリエーションルーム Recreation Room　④ 廊下 Hallway

千壽介護老人保健施設
Senju Geriatric Health Care Services Facility

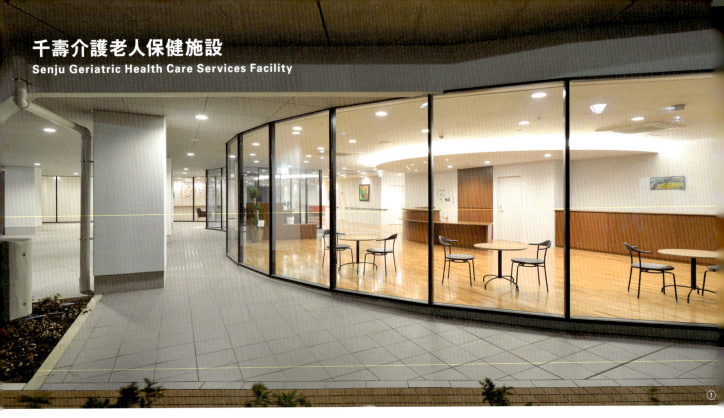

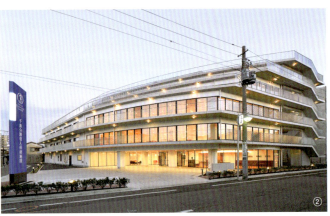

かつて千住宿とよばれ、江戸時代には日光街道・奥州街道の一番目の宿場として栄えた地域に建ち、大きな窓が印象的な、明るく開放感のある施設。フロアーごとにキッチンを備えた広々としたダイニングルームを配し、家庭的な雰囲気で食事をすることができる。

The Senju facility is located in an area previously called Senju-shu-ku, which prospered during the Edo period (1600-1868) as the first station along the Nikko Kaido and Oshu Kaido, important routes that connected Edo (now Tokyo) to other important locations. The facility's impressively large windows create a cheery and open feeling. Spacious dining rooms with kitchens are on each floor, so that guests can enjoy their meals in a homey atmosphere.

千壽グループホーム
Senju Group Home

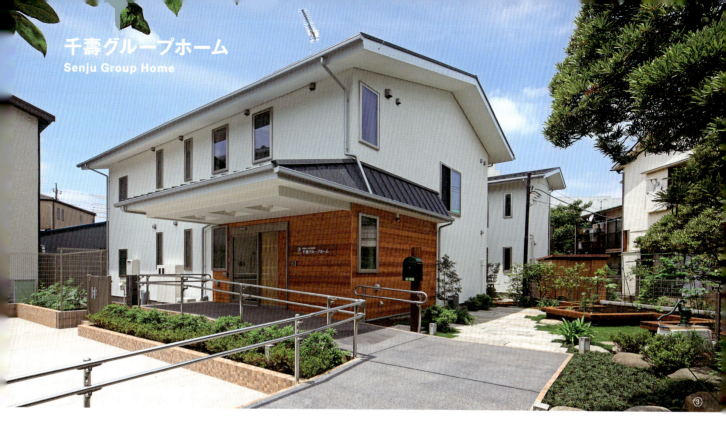

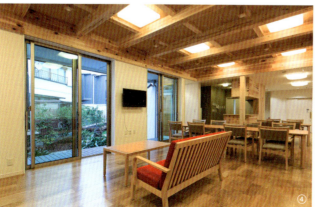

千壽介護老人保健施設
入所（短期含む）：148 名
通所リハビリ：36 名
施設：4人室、2人室、個室
〒120-0035
東京都足立区千住中居町 29-6
TEL. 03-5284-0088

Senju Geriatric Health Care Services Facility
Long-stay & short-stay: 148 guests
Day-care (rehabilitation): 36 guests
Type of rooms: Four-person, double, and private
29-6 Senjunakaicho, Adachi-ku, Tokyo 120-0035
Tel.: 03-5284-0088

千壽グループホーム
入所：18 名
〒120-0035
東京都足立区千住中居町 30-3
TEL. 03-3879-0088

Senju Group Home
Long-stay: 18 guests
30-3 Senjunakaicho,
Adachi-ku, Tokyo 120-0035
Tel.: 03-3879-0088

① エントランス夜景 Entrance night view ② 外観 Exterior view
③ グループホーム外観 Exterior of Group Home
④ グループホームのリビングルーム Living room of Group Home

ワセダグループホーム
Waseda Group Home

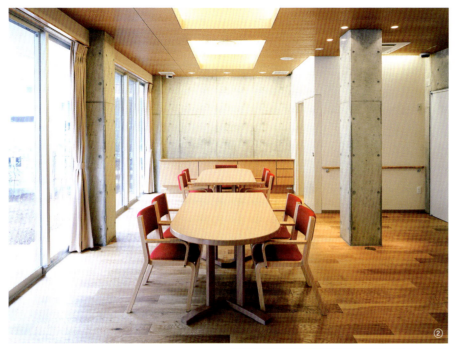
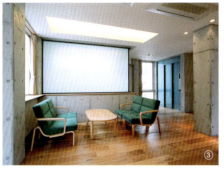
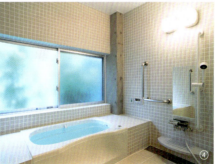
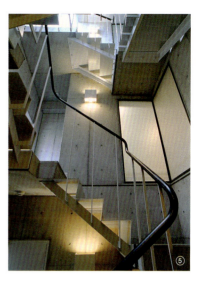

ワセダグループホーム
入所：9名
〒162-0041
東京都新宿区早稲田鶴巻町 519-3
TEL. 03-5292-0088

Waseda Group Home
Long-stay: 9 guests
519-3 Wasedatsurumakicho, Shinjuku-ku, Tokyo 162-0041
Tel.: 03-5292-0088

認知症のゲストが、その人らしく生活できるよう配慮された施設。掃除や洗濯、食事の支度、散歩など、家庭と同じような日常生活を送ることで、ゲストの安心感を高めている。家庭的なスケールのリビングや食堂、浴室を備え、スタッフたちの温かいケアーが受けられる。

The Waseda facility helps guests suffering from dementia to lead lives with human dignity. Leading everyday lives of cleaning, doing laundry, preparing meals, and going for walks, guests are able to feel safe and secure. Guests are provided with a family-sized living room, dining room, and bathroom, and receive the staff's warm-hearted care.

① 外観 Exterior view
② リビングルーム Living Room
③ 談話コーナー Conversation Corner
④ 浴室 Bathroom
⑤ 階段室 Stairwell

青葉ヒルズ(特別養護老人ホーム)
Aoba Hills (Special Nursing Home)

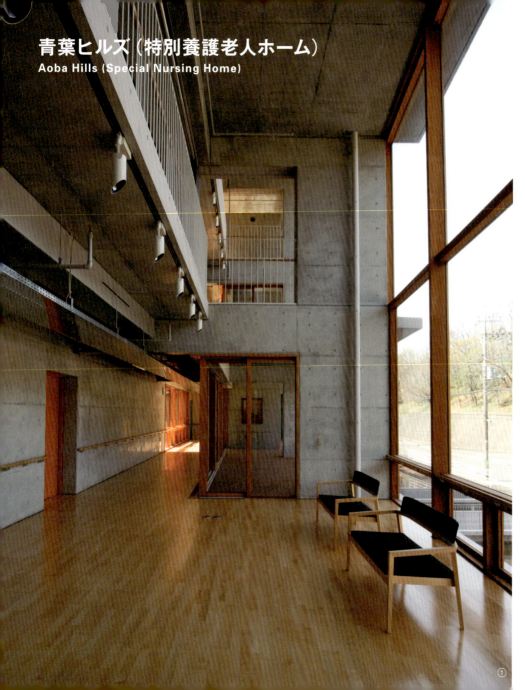

2007年12月に設立した社会福祉法人龍岡会によるひとつ目の施設。緑豊かな丘陵地にあり、外観、インテリア共に天然の木材を多く使うことで、周囲の環境に溶け込む施設となっている。10室ごとにユニットを構成し、家庭的な雰囲気のケアーを行っている。

Aoba Hills is the first facility of Medical Corporation Tatsuoka, which was established in December 2007. Located in the hilly green countryside, the facility's natural wood exterior and interior make it beautifully adapted to its environment. Aoba Hills has ten rooms per unit and provides nursing care in a family-like environment.

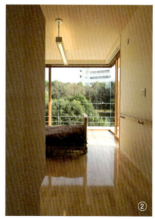

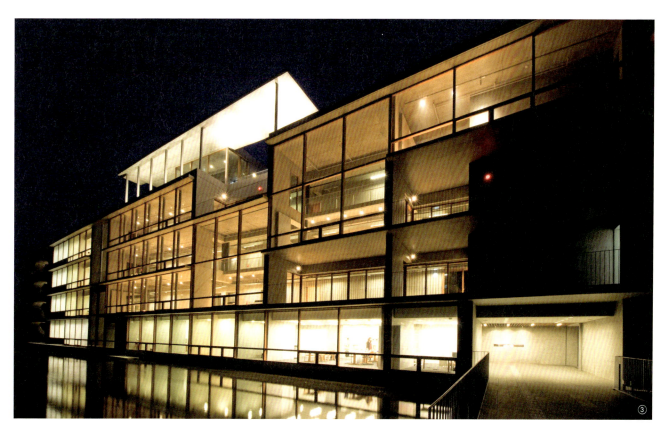

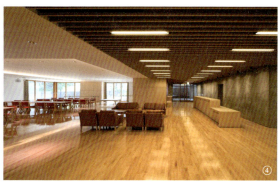

青葉ヒルズ（特別養護老人ホーム）
入所：120 名
ショートステイ：20 名
通所介護：10 名
施設：個室
〒227-0033
神奈川県横浜市青葉区鴨志田町 1260
TEL. 045-961-0088

Aoba Hills (Special Nursing Home)
Long-stay: 120 guests
Short-stay: 20 guests
Day-care: 10 guests
Type of rooms: Private
1260 Kamoshidacho, Aoba-ku,
Yokohama-shi, Kanagawa 227-0033
Tel.: 045-961-0088

① ラウンジ Lounge ② 個室 Private room
③ 外観夜景 Exterior night view ④ エントランスロビー Entrance Lobby

龍岡会 施設設計者・施工者 一覧

龍岡介護老人保健施設
設計：黒川雅之建築設計事務所　施工：清水建設

浅草介護老人保健施設
設計：黒川雅之建築設計事務所　施工：竹中工務店

櫻川介護老人保健施設
設計：黒川雅之建築設計事務所　施工：安藤建設

神石介護老人保健施設
設計：千代田設計　施工：大木建設

千壽介護老人保健施設
設計：黒川紀章建築都市設計事務所　施工：清水建設

千壽グループホーム
設計：ちち建築設計工房　施工：鈴木工務店

ワセダグループホーム
設計：黒川雅之建築設計事務所　施工：大木建設

青葉ヒルズ（特別養護老人ホーム）
設計：野生司環境設計　施工：りんかい日産建設・石井建設

写真クレジット
新 良太　P36、P39、P134-135
土田有里子　P88
タテルデザイン　P120左上
濱津和貴　P120左下
黒川未来夫　P85、P126-127、P130、P132-133
坂田峰夫　P128-129
清水 昭　P24、P59、P122-125
hanafactory　P131

龍岡会の考える
介護のあたりまえ
豊かに生きる、地域で暮らす

2016年8月8日　初版第一刷発行
著：大森順方
ブックデザイン：岩松亮太
編集・取材協力：殿井悠子（オフィスノベンタ）
イラスト・オブジェ制作：田中靖夫
発行：建築画報社
160-0022 東京都新宿区新宿 2-14-6 第一早川屋ビル
TEL 03-3356-2568
www.kenchiku-gahou.com

定価：2,400円（税別）

印刷・製本：北斗社

乱丁・落丁本はお取り替えいたします　無断で本書の全体または一部の複写・複製をすることを禁じます
©2016 龍岡会 ALL rights reserved　Printed in Japan 978-4-901772-92-1

Designers and Builders of the Tatsuoka Group Facilities

Tatsuoka Geriatric Health Care Services Facility
Design: K-Studio (Masayuki Kurosawa)　Construction: Shimizu Corporation

Asakusa Geriatric Health Care Services Facility
Design: K-Studio (Masayuki Kurosawa)　Construction: Takenaka Corporation

Sakuragawa Geriatric Health Care Services Facility
Design: K-Studio (Masayuki Kurosawa)　Construction: Ando Corporation

Kamiishi Geriatric Health Care Services Facility
Design: Chiyoda Architects & Engineers' Office　Construction: Ohki Corporation

Senju Geriatric Health Care Services Facility
Design: Kisho Kurokawa architect & associates　Construction: Shimizu Corporation

Senju Group Home
Design: Chichi Architects' Design Studio　Construction: Suzuki Komuten

Waseda Group Home
Design: K-Studio (Masayuki Kurosawa)　Construction: Ohki Corporation

Aoba Hills (Special Nursing Home)
Design: Nosu Architects Planners Engineers
Construction: Rinkai Construction Co., Ltd. / Ishii Kensetsu

Photography Credits
Ryota Atarashi: P36, P39, P134-135
Yuriko Tsuchida: P88
TaTel Design: P120 top left
Waki Hamatsu: P120 bottom left
Mikio Kurokawa: P85, P126-127, P130, P132-133
Mineo Sakata: P128-129
Akira Shimizu: P24, P59, P122-125
hanafactory: P131

Tatsuoka Group's
Standard in Human Care

A Rich, Full Life, Lived in the Community

August 8, 2016　First edition, first printing
Author: Nobumasa Ohmori
Book design: Ryota Iwamatsu
Editing and research assistance: Chikako Tonoi (noventa)
Illustration and creation of curios: Yasuo Tanaka
Publisher: Kenchiku Gahou Inc.
2-14-6 Shinjuku, Shinjuku-ku, Tokyo 160-0022
TEL 03-3356-2568
www.kenchiku-gahou.com

Retail Price: 2,400 yen(+tax)

Printing and binding: Hokutosha